International Cooperation for Registration of Medicines

TEAM LEADER

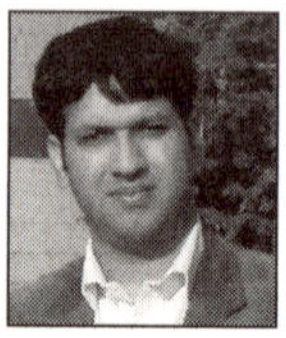

Ali Mehdi established and leads the Health Policy Initiative at ICRIER. His research interests include—the process, design and assessment of health policies; prevention of chronic diseases along with policy instruments and institutional design for its promotion; social determinants of health; metrics of health inequities; health financing, governance and manpower; fertility and mortality; demographic dividend; drug regulation. A couple of his books are in the pipeline—*India Health Report 2018* (Oxford University Press), *A Shot of Justice* (2 volumes) (Oxford University Press), *Chronic Diseases in South Asia* (Springer), *Freedoms and Fragility: The Challenge of Job Creation in Kashmir, India* (Routledge). Ali did his MA at the University of Freiburg, Germany and completed his PhD at Humboldt University in Berlin. He can be reached at *amehdi@icrier.res.in*.

AUTHORS

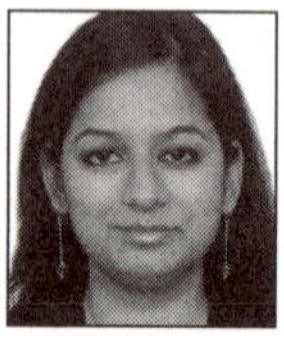

Vasudha Wattal is a Research Associate at ICRIER, and has been associated with the Health Policy Initiative since its inception in 2014. She is specifically involved in the drug regulatory project and has contributed to various publications developed under this research program. She has also co-authored a number of opinion pieces and journal articles on several policy issues such as drug regulation, economics of drug pricing and air pollution. Her research interests include, economics of competition, economics of health and behavioural economics. Vasudha holds a Masters and an M.Phil. Degree in Economics.

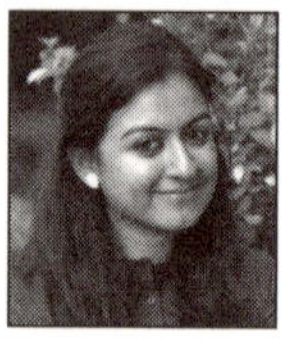

Pallavi Joshi is a Research Associate at ICRIER, and is working on governance and regulatory aspects of healthcare sector and pharmaceutical industry, for publications under Health Policy Initiative. Previously, she has worked with Competition Commission of India, where she was involved in analysing competition issues in various sectors, in particular—healthcare sector, and pharmaceutical industry. She has also worked with Standard & Poor's Capital IQ, a business research firm. Her core areas of interest include development economics, health economics, pharmaceutical regulation, behavioural economics, and competition law. She holds a Masters degree in Economics.

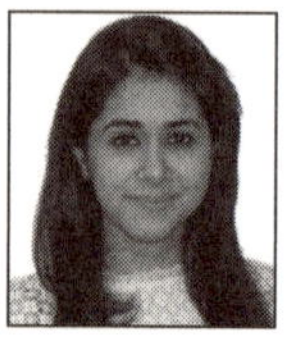

Aashna Arora is a Consultant at ICRIER under the Health Policy Initiative. Her interest areas include health economics, environmental economics, trade and economics, public policy and ethics in policymaking. She has a passion to work for policy oriented research on issues that impact public health and access to health and medicines in India. Previously, she has worked at KPMG as a Business Associate in the Research, Analysis and Knowledge unit and interned with the Ministry of Health and Family Welfare. She holds a Masters degree in Economics.

International Cooperation for Registration of Medicines

Opportunities for India

Team Leader
Ali Mehdi

Authors
Vasudha Wattal
Pallavi Joshi
Aashna Arora

ACADEMIC FOUNDATION
NEW DELHI

www.academicfoundation.org

First published in 2017
by

ACADEMIC FOUNDATION
4772-73 / 23 Bharat Ram Road, (23 Ansari Road),
Darya Ganj, New Delhi - 110 002 (India).
Phones : 23245001 / 02.
Fax : +91-11-23245005.
E-mail : booksaf@gmail.com
www.academicfoundation.org

and

INDIAN COUNCIL FOR RESEARCH ON INTERNATIONAL ECONOMIC RELATIONS (ICRIER)
Core 6A, 4th Floor India Habitat Centre, Lodhi Road, New Delhi 110003

Disclaimer: Opinions and recommendations in the report are exclusively of the author(s) and not of any other individual or institution including ICRIER. This report has been prepared in good faith on the basis of information available at the date of publication. All interactions and transactions with industry sponsors and their representatives have been transparent and conducted in an open, honest and independent manner as enshrined in ICRIER Memorandum of Association. ICRIER does not accept any corporate funding that comes with a mandated research area which is not in line with ICRIER's research agenda. The corporate funding of an ICRIER activity does not, in any way, imply ICRIER's endorsement of the views of the sponsoring organization or its products or policies. ICRIER does not conduct research that is focused on any specific product or service provided by the corporate sponsor.

Citation:
Wattal, V., Joshi, P., Arora, A., Mehdi, A.* (2017). *International cooperation for registration of medicines: Opportunities for India*. New Delhi: Academic Foundation.
(*: Corresponding Author: *amehdi@icrier.res.in*)

Cataloging in Publication Data--DK
Courtesy: D.K. Agencies (P) Ltd. <docinfo@dkagencies.com>

Mehdi, Ali, author.
International cooperation for registration of medicines : opportunities for India.
pages cm
Includes bibliographical references.
ISBN 9789332704251

1. Drug registration–India. 2. Drug registration–International cooperation. 3. Medical policy–India. I. Wattal, Vasudha, author. II. Joshi, Pallavi, author. III. Arora, Aashna, author. IV. Indian Council for Research on International Economic Relations, issuing body. V. Title.

KNS1536.M44 2017 DDC 344.540423 23

Typeset, printed and bound by The Book Mint, New Delhi.
www.thebookmint.in

Contents

List of Tables, Figures and Appendix

Tables

Figures

Appendix

List of Abbreviations

API	Active Pharmaceutical Ingredient
ADR	Adverse Drug Reactions
AMRH	African Medicines Regulatory Harmonization
ANDA	Abbreviated NDA
ASEAN	Association of South-East Asian Nations
ACCSQ	ASEAN Consultative Committee for Standards and Quality
ACTD	ASEAN Common Technical Document
ACTR	ASEAN Common Technical Requirements
APRIA	ASEAN Pharmaceutical Research Industry Associations
APC	ASEAN Pharmaceutical Club
APEC	Asia Pacific Economic Cooperation
AFTA	ASEAN Free Trade Area
BABE	Bioavailability and Bioequivalence
BE	Bioequivalence
BCS	Biopharmaceutics Classification System
BLA	Biologic Drug Application
CDSCO	Central Drugs Standard Control Organization
CDL	Central Drugs Laboratory
CFDA	China Food and Drug Administration
CHMP	Committee for Medicinal Products for Human Use
CIOMS	Council for International Organizations of Medical Sciences
CTD	Common Technical Document
CECA	Comprehensive Economic Cooperation Agreement
COPP	Certificate of Pharmaceutical Product
CBER	Centre for Biologics Evaluation and Research
CDER	Centre for Drug Evaluation and Research
CMS	Concerned Member States
CMD(h)	Coordination Group for Mutual Recognition and Decentralised Procedures for Human Medicinal Products
COO	Country of Origin
CP	Centralised Procedure
CPMP	Committee for Proprietary Medicinal Products
CoRE	Centre of Regulatory Excellence
CTD	Common Technical Document
DCA	Drugs and Cosmetics Act, 1940
DCR	Drugs and Cosmetic Rules, 1945
DCGI	Drugs Controller General of India
DCP	Decentralised Procedure
DGHS	Director-General of Health Services
DRA	Drug Regulatory Authorities
DTAB	Drugs Technical Advisory Board
DPCO	Drugs Prices Control Order
EAC	East African Community
ECs	Ethics Committees
eCTD	electronic Common Technical Document
EDL	Essential Drug List
EMA	European Medicines Agency
EU	European Union
EUDRA	European Union Drug Regulatory Authorities
FDA	Food and Drug Administration
FDASIA	Food and Drug Administration Safety and Innovation Act
FRPs	Facilitated Regulatory Pathways
GCP	Good Clinical Practice

GDA	Generic Drug Application
GDP	Gross Domestic Product
GDUFA	Generic Drug User Fee Act
GMP	Good Manufacturing Practices
HSA	Health Sciences Authority
HPA	Health Products Act
HPRG	Health Products Regulation Group
IND	Investigational New Drug
ICH	International Council on Harmonisation of Technical Requirements for Registration of Pharmaceuticals for Human Use
ICMRA	International Coalition of Medicines Regulatory Authorities
IGDRP	International Generic Drug Regulators Programme
LMICs	Low and Middle Income Countries
MCC	Medical Control Council
MDGs	Millennium Development Goals
MHRA	Medicines and Healthcare Products Regulatory
MNCs	Multinational Companies
MRA	Mutual Recognition Agreement
MRP	Mutual Recognition Procedure
MRFG	Mutual Recognition Facilitation Group
MoU	Memorandum of Understanding
MoHFW	Ministry of Health and Family Welfare
NADFC	National Agency of Drug and Food Control
NCE	New Chemical Entity
NCDs	Non-communicable Diseases
NDA	New Drug Application
NEPAD	New Partnership for Africa's Development
NOC	No Objection Certificate
NPA	National Pharmaceutical Administration
NTB	Non-tariff Barriers
PANDRH	Pan American Network on Drug Regulatory Harmonization
PAP	Pan African Parliament
PDUFA	Prescription Drug User Fee Act
PIC/S	Pharmaceutical Inspections Co-operation Scheme
PPWG	Pharmaceuticals Product Working Group
PRIME	PRIority MEdicines
PRISM	Pharmaceutical Regulatory Information System
REC	Regional Economic Communities
RMS	Reference Member State
SADC	Southern African Development Community
SC	Steering Committee
SDGs	Sustainable Development Goals
SDRA	State Drug Regulatory Authority
SEC	Subject Expert Committee
SAHPRA	South African Health Products Regulatory Authority
SIAHR	Supporting the Implementation of ASEAN Harmonized Requirements for Drug Registration
SMEs	Small and Medium Enterprises
SND	Subsequent New Drug
TP	Therapeutic Products
TRIPS	Trade Related Aspects of Intellectual Property Rights
US	United States
USFDA	United States Food and Drug Administration
WHO	World Health Organization

Foreword

As India tackles its triple burden of disease, the demand for newer and better medicines—safe, effective and of prescribed quality—needs to be adequately addressed. This will not be possible without efficient drug registration processes that have the potential to minimise delays in access to timely medical interventions. The Indian pharmaceutical industry has established itself as a global leader in the pharmaceutical space, and it is the right time for Indian drug regulators to step up their participation in relevant international forums, contributing as well as learning to fulfil their mandate of protecting and promoting public health in India—as well as globally.

This report analyses some of the major ongoing initiatives of international cooperation for drug registration and explores policy options for the Government of India with a focus on addressing its burden of disease as well as promotion of the Indian pharmaceutical industry. India is widely seen as a global leader—India's drug regulators too should prepare for a proactive global role, to learn and contribute as best as they can, with a focus on local as well as global public health.

I hope all stakeholders—particularly policymakers in the Government of India, representatives of pharmaceutical industry, civil society, international organisations and academia find this report interesting and stimulating.

— Rajat Kathuria
Director and Chief Executive
Indian Council for Research on International Economic Relations (ICRIER)
New Delhi

Acknowledgements

Conducting the comprehensive and analytical nature of research that we have been under the Health Policy Initiative (HPI) at ICRIER since 2014 would not have been possible without the generous and unconditional financial support provided by the Pharmaceutical Research and Manufacturers of America (PhRMA), Washington DC. We would, therefore, like to, first and foremost, thank PhRMA in general and Ms Amiee Aloi, Deputy Vice President of International Advocacy at PhRMA in particular for such support—and more importantly, for an independent think-tank like ICRIER, their supportive attitude towards our nonpartisan approach.

As part of our nonpartisan approach, we, at HPI, adopted a strong stakeholder orientation from the beginning. All topics of research, and their scope, were decided based on discussions during two multistakeholder workshops in early 2014. Since then, we have maintained this orientation and we would like to thank all stakeholders,in India and abroad, who participated in this study and made it possible—during the course of various consultations, one-to-one meetings, etc.

We have been privileged to have some of the most renowned national and international experts in the field to review this study and offer their insightful comments for improvement. Mr Mark Barnes and Dr Barbara Bierer of the prestigious Multiregional Clinical Trials Center (MRCT) at Harvard University, USA; Mr Richard Kingham, Senior Counsel, Covington & Burling LLP in Washington, DC/London as well as Adjunct Professor at the Georgetown University Law Centre, USA; Ms Susan Winckler, President of Leavitt Partners Consulting, Washington, DC, USA; Mr Andy Gray, Senior Lecturer, Division of Pharmacology, School of Health Sciences, University of KwaZulu-Natal, South Africa; Dr B.K. Rana, CEO Incharge, National Accreditation Board for Hospitals and Healthcare Providers (NABH), New Delhi; Dr Santanu Tripathi, Professor and Head, Department of Clinical and Experimental Pharmacology, Calcutta School of Tropical Medicine, Kolkata and Mr D.G. Shah, Secretary General of the Indian Pharmaceutical Alliance (IPA), Mumbai deserve special mention in this regard.

Our special thanks are due to highly distinguished members of the Advisory Committee of our Research Program on Drug Regulatory Reforms in India. We benefited immensely from their guidance and support throughout the process of this study. We would like to thank Richard and Susan in particular for travelling all the way from Washington, DC to participate in the Advisory Committee meetings.

Finally—and most importantly—I would like to express my profoundest gratitude to Dr Rajat Kathuria, Director and CE, ICRIER and my HPI colleagues, who worked with great dedication and put out their best at various stages of this study. All credit goes to them, while I take responsibility for any shortcomings that remain.

This acknowledgement would not be complete without thanking Mr Sanu Kapila and Ms Sona Kapila at Academic Foundation for promptly agreeing, preparing and bringing out this report in such a professional manner. A big thank you to them and their team!

—Ali Mehdi
Fellow and Project Leader
Health Policy Initiative
Indian Council for Research on International Economic Relations (ICRIER), New Delhi
email: amehdi@icrier.res.in

Executive Summary

There has been a great deal of international interaction and cooperation in the area of public health, particularly since the conception of the Millennium Development Goals (MDGs). However, while world leaders agreed upon and signed a specific set of health goals and targets as part of the MDGs, and recently under the Sustainable Development Goals (SDGs)—which are to be achieved by 2030—international cooperation vis-à-vis mechanisms to achieve those shared goals is still very limited. Regulation of medicines/drugs is one of them. Drug regulation aims at protecting and promoting public health by establishing the safety, efficacy and quality of medicines. Despite commonalities in the science and objectives of regulation, drug regulatory authorities differ significantly in their respective requirements and capacities, contributing to inequalities in access to medicines as well as health outcomes across nations. Such a realisation has inspired a number of efforts to minimise divergences and pool the capacities of national regulators.

In India, the need for an efficient and easier drug registration process assumes greater significance in the backdrop of rapidly changing pattern of diseases—requiring newer and better treatments—and the pharmaceutical industry increasingly involved in drug innovation/discovery. This study—the first of its kind—seeks to identify key areas of concern in the process of medicine registration in India and the supportive role that international cooperation can play in this context. It reviews some of the major international cooperation initiatives for registration of medicines to identify lessons as well as opportunities that the Government of India could potentially leverage to address its regulatory challenges and achieve the goals of public health in particular. Although there are a range of economic and political factors that impact access to medicines in a country, this study focuses on institutional factors that have a bearing on regulatory processes related to registration.

1

Introduction

There has been a great deal of international interaction and cooperation in the area of public health, particularly since the conception of the MDGs. However, while world leaders agreed upon and signed a specific set of health goals and targets as part of the MDGs, and recently under the SDGs—which are to be achieved by 2030—international cooperation vis-à-vis mechanisms to achieve those shared goals is still very limited. Regulation of medicines/drugs is one of them.[1] Drug regulation aims at protecting and promoting public health by establishing the safety, efficacy, and quality of medicines. Despite commonalities in the science and objectives of regulation, drug regulatory authorities (DRAs) differ significantly in their respective requirements and capacities, contributing to inequalities in access to medicines as well as health outcomes across nations. Such a realisation has inspired several efforts to minimise divergences and pool the capacities of national regulators. International cooperation initiatives also promote ease of doing business for an increasingly global pharmaceutical industry and enhance the attractiveness of initiatives like 'Make in India'.

Figure 1.1

Stages of Regulatory Approvals in the Process of Drug Development

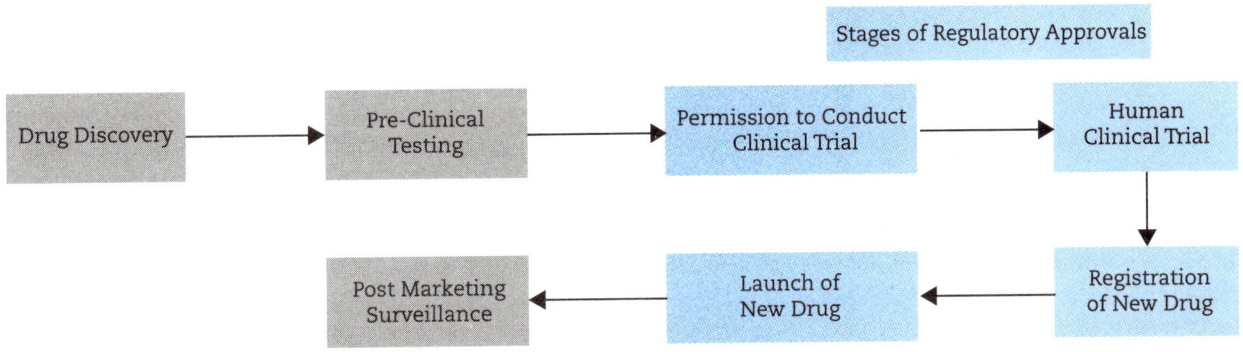

Note: The blue boxes represent stages of regulatory intervention.

Source: Developed by authors.

Drug registration is a critical step for the introduction of a medicine in a country (refer to Figure 1.1 for the steps involved in drug development and the stages requiring regulatory approvals). The process starts with the submission of a dossier by a company to the regulator and culminates in approval/rejection and subsequent registration of the final product on the basis of an assessment of safety, quality and efficacy parameters of the drug. Various international cooperation initiatives have facilitated pathways to streamline the submission and review processes. The International Council for Harmonisation of Technical Requirements for Pharmaceuticals for Human Use (ICH) and Association of Southeast Asian Nations (ASEAN), for instance, have developed a common dossier format—the ICH/ASEAN Common Technical Document (CTD)—although subsequent review and registration processes are still national. A CTD is a shared template, which can potentially form the basis for review interactions among various national regulators. Alternatively, developing countries have also sought to learn from each other through a shared review process—for example ZAZIBONA[2]—which enables them to bridge gaps through leveraging their respective regulatory capacities as well as draw collectively from more sophisticated international regulators.

This study aims to develop policy recommendations for addressing key challenges associated with registration of medicines in the Indian context. To do so, it reviews some of the major international cooperation initiatives for registration of medicines to identify lessons as well as opportunities that the Government of India could potentially leverage to address its regulatory challenges and achieve the goals of public health. Although there are a range of economic and political factors that impact access to medicines in a country, this study focuses on institutional factors that have a bearing on the

1. Throughout this report, 'drug' refers to new chemical entities (NCEs), generics and biosimilars. For the purpose of this study, the term drug is used for medicinal products intended for human use, and is used interchangeably with medicine, pharmaceutical product and pharmaceuticals.

2. ZAZIBONA is collaboration between DRAs of Botswana, Namibia, Zambia, Zimbabwe, and South Africa to conduct joint assessments.

regulatory processes related to medicine registration. Technical standards of safety, quality, and efficacy are matters of scientific expertise and, thus, beyond the scope of a policy study like ours.

1.1 Importance of the Subject—Rationale

Drug regulators in developing countries like India are heavily constrained if we consider their roles in the backdrop of the massive burden of disease, disability, and premature mortality and the limited human, technical, and financial resources at their disposal. A highly rational and efficient utilisation of existing resources is the only option available to them. Rather than reinvent the wheel, regulators can explore best practices from around the world, cooperate with, and leverage capacities of other regulators wherever required, with an eye on addressing our own health and regulatory challenges. For example, developed regulatory authorities have extensive experience in assessment of NCEs, while their counterparts in developing countries face considerable challenges in processing newer and complex data due to capacity constraints (Gray 2004, DFID 2004). This is one of the areas where the latter can leverage the international experience. At the same time, the latter can engage in and influence international decision-making and standard-setting in areas where they may have comparative advantage. International cooperation works to mutual advantage, and that is how it needs to be viewed by policymakers/regulators.

'Unnecessary differences'[3] in regulations—as Cecilia Malmström, European Commission's Trade Commissioner (2014-2019) argued—are a 'significant barrier' to open markets, more growth, and more jobs. Regulators should strike a balance between 'protection' (based on what is scientifically valid and needed) and 'promotion' (by proactively fostering the forces) of public health. With increasing globalisation of the pharmaceutical industry—not least of Indian origin—regulators can no longer promote public health by means of an inward-looking attitude—they need to connect and cooperate with counterparts in other countries and make best use of their limited resources. An international regulatory outreach should also match up with the country's increasing involvement and stature at the world stage as well as its international commitments, particularly in the area of health. India's drug regulatory framework should no longer be out of sync with either the country's public health challenges—requiring a proactive outreach—or its broader political economy.

At the same time, in exploring the most relevant routes for international cooperation in medicine registration, it is important to appreciate country specificities. Challenges in medicine registration in developed and developing countries are not always alike. International cooperation depends on several factors, including size and nature of market for medicinal products (generics, NCEs). As a one-size-fits-all approach does not work, the present study uses a game theoretic model[4] to explain the pay-offs for various stakeholders from international cooperation in drug registration. As such, it puts forth potential ways in which India can have a more robust and efficient drug registration process and participate in ongoing international cooperation initiatives to its advantage. Our public health and related resource challenges are enormous—but so are the opportunities to address them by making the most rational and efficient use of our limited resources and leveraging international resources to our best advantage.

1.2 Major Pathways of International Cooperation for Registration of Medicines

The creation of the European Union (EU) and a European market provided the first and most significant impetus towards international drug regulatory cooperation. Europe's central drug approval policies aimed at improving the welfare of consumers and producers alike (Vogel 1998). EU integration efforts, and later ICH, have made harmonisation the most widely prevalent pattern of collaboration among regulators. Harmonisation is a step-by-step process, which involves repeated consultations between participating countries over a range of regulatory procedures, including drug registration and related safety, quality and efficacy guidelines. It is often argued that harmonisation borrows from the language of trade agreements. However, several respondents in our field research

3. Speech of Cecilia Malmström, Commissioner for Trade, European Commission, 19 March 2015. Available at *http://trade.ec.europa.eu/doclib/docs/2015/march/tradoc_153260.pdf* (Last accessed on 13 April 2017).

4. A game theoretic model uses mathematics to explain decision-making behaviour for two or more players who face alternate strategies, either simultaneously or sequentially. The outcomes from such strategic decision-making critically relies on the payoffs resulting from these interdependent strategies. In the current context, game theoretic model is used to explain the rationale for countries in making optimal strategic choices for participation in international cooperation initiatives.

suggested that the latter should be treated as separate from the former, especially in the context of medicine registration. This is because while trade agreements bind countries to work together for a certain output, harmonisation relates to working together to come up with a template of standard procedures. Nonetheless, in order to give it a more 'politically palatable' tone and address concerns over national sovereignty, 'regulatory convergence'[5] has emerged as a more acceptable concept in policy circles. Convergence is a broader concept of international cooperation among regulatory authorities such that each attains the same level of standards in the long run.[6] It is important to note here that convergence does not require the harmonisation of different countries' laws and regulations,[7] and yet opens up possibilities for additional, enhanced forms of cooperation and collaboration between regulatory authorities. The ongoing efforts towards achieving regulatory convergence in pharmaceuticals appear more in the nature of a semi-voluntary process.[8] For instance, the approach of the Pan American Network for Drug Regulatory Harmonisation (PANDRH) and Asia-Pacific Economic Cooperation (APEC) is such that regulatory requirements across economies or countries become more aligned over time, following from the adoption of internationally recognised technical guidance, standards and best practices. The International Generic Drug Regulators Programme (IGDRP) is also aimed at regulatory convergence and cooperation in the review of generic drug applications across participating nations by establishing a more permanent information and work-sharing arrangement.[9]

Streamlining regulatory procedures can also be achieved through mutual recognition agreements (MRAs). MRAs are bilateral/multilateral agreements among countries that seek to promote trade and facilitate market access by lowering technical barriers to trade. MRAs work on the principle of mutual recognition, with participating nations agreeing to recognise each other's conformity assessments, including testing, certificates, product standards, etc.[10] Mutual recognition could be an outcome of several elements, including a harmonised set of guidelines developed by participating countries, an equivalence agreement or external criteria like international standards or importing countries' standards (TACD 2001).

Regulatory convergence is linked and yet distinct from other pathways such as harmonisation and MRAs. While harmonisation is not a prerequisite for regulatory convergence, but once harmonised standards have been adopted by a group of nations, convergence of processes as well as outcomes between them is expected to follow. Mutual recognition is also capable of driving regulatory convergence and is a relatively easy process that requires fewer resources and commitment. However, there may be challenges in achieving this when there are asymmetries in regulatory systems, approaches and cultures among participating nations. MRAs can work when participating countries have comparable and mutually agreeable regulatory capacities. If there are substantial capacity differences, there is usually a unilateral system of recognition where relatively stronger regulatory agencies are considered as reference points by smaller countries. A number of developing country regulators have adopted the latter to overcome their regulatory limitations by relying on the expertise and judgment of developed country regulators. It also happens informally at a broader scale where the former rely on the latter for specific cases rather than generally.

1.3 Need for India to Respond from a Public Health Perspective

As discussed, various patterns of international cooperation for registration of medicines have

5. Regulatory convergence refers to the growing similarity of three elements—institutional frameworks, policy approaches and outcomes in the regulatory politics. The process of convergence is dynamic and catalysed by workload, globalisation, technology, and public expectations and that way it considers disparate capabilities. See more at: Falkner and Gupta (2009).

6. See Lustig and Weisfeld (2013).

7. Ibid.

8. Regulatory convergence can be voluntary; semi-voluntary or mandatory. Voluntary convergence can be market induced or spontaneously inspired by the legal practices of other countries. On the other hand, semi-voluntary and mandatory convergence can be attributed to the activities of international standard setting organisations (intergovernmental or non-governmental). Semi voluntary convergence differs from mandatory convergence in that, the former may be initiated through instruments of "soft law", which may be transposed into domestic laws by the concerned regulatory authorities and eventually become mandatory, whereas in the latter, participation in international organisations automatically implies the compulsory acceptance of the norms enacted by these organisations. More at: Stephanou (2003).

9. See *http://www.who.int/medicines/publications/druginformation/DI_28-1_Regulatory-Harmonization.pdf* (Last accessed on 13 April 2017).

10. The cost of conformity assessment could be substantial, especially for products that are required to be tested, both prior to export and at the port of entry. See, Swann (2010).

been explored by countries, both developed and developing, in several parts of the world. However, India presently does not proactively participate in any international cooperation initiative.[11] There are a number of questions which have been raised in this regard—for instance, why should Indian regulators worry about international cooperation? How does the country stand to benefit from such cooperation? What cost would such cooperation entail for various stakeholders? Given our rapidly changing disease profile, requiring newer and better treatment, and the increasing global profile of Indian pharmaceutical industry, we need to consider and address questions like these on a priority basis. There should be no anxieties attached to such discussion if we take a considered view of the cooperation initiatives around the world. This is what this report particularly aims at—to facilitate a rational discussion and consideration of international cooperation for registration of medicines in the context of our public health and economic considerations in particular. However, it needs to be clarified here that, from a purely drug regulatory perspective, the consideration of public health should be assigned priority over all else in the discussion of international cooperation.

As elaborated in the pages that follow, international cooperation has different meanings to different regulatory contexts. From the vantage point of benefits to public health, international cooperation can be seen as a tool to foster faster accessibility and availability of quality medicines. Towards this end, various international forums like IGDRP, ICH, ZAZIBONA initiative, WHO Prequalification Programme, etc. are good examples of increasing access and availability of medicines through international cooperation. Such platforms could be learning opportunities for resource-constrained developing countries in strengthening their national regulatory systems. Further, even in broad areas of health policy, international collaboration is seen as a way forward. With respect to achieving SDGs in particular, there is a global push towards building partnerships as countries work towards building capacities to address health challenges within a cooperative framework. Different avenues and forums for the achievement of international health goals should be explored—international cooperation for registration of medicines being a potentially important one. While international cooperation alone should not be expected to completely solve the problem of access to medicines, it could significantly contribute to—possibilities of systemised/facilitated routes of medicine registration, enhanced access to markets resulting in more legitimate business that brings in registered medicines and weeds out fake or substandard ones in the domestic market, efficient utilisation of regulatory resources by reduction of duplicative processes—highlight a few that emerged from our expert interactions. Given that we are the world's biggest contributor to premature deaths—both at the child (under 5 years) and adult (between 30 and 70 years) levels (Mehdi et al. 2016)—we need to explore and discuss everything on earth that can help us address such a colossal waste of human life and resource. Given our rising international stature, particularly in recent years, there is nothing that should keep us away from international participation, cooperation—and leadership. Policy hesitation is not going to solve our public health problems (it hasn't until now)—confidently considering and addressing them surely will.

This report is divided into seven chapters. Chapter 2 discusses the research methodology. Chapter 3 presents an analysis of the issues in the drug registration process in India and select countries. Chapter 4 presents cross-country impact assessments of international cooperation initiatives from the perspective of public health, industry and regulators. Chapter 5 contains discussion of international cooperation as a coordination game. Based on analyses in the preceding chapters, a list of policy recommendations for the Indian context have been drawn up, which are presented in Chapter 6. Finally, the conclusions are presented in Chapter 7.

11. It, however, may be noted that India now is one of the ICH observers, and stands to gain from the deliberations.

2

Research Methodology

In order to examine the role of international cooperation initiatives in a global context and subsequently analyse the impact for various stakeholders in India, both desk and field research were conducted. The former was carried out through a survey of existing academic literature along with governmental and inter-governmental reports, data from websites of regulatory authorities and international forums, journal articles, etc. This was followed up with semi-structured interviews across a range of stakeholders in national and selected international jurisdictions for cross-country comparisons. Stakeholder categories included regulators (Central Drugs Standard Control Organization [CDSCO] and its counterparts in other international jurisdictions), industry (representatives from small/medium/large industry segments as well as Multinational Companies (MNCs)), civil society (patient advocacy groups, procurement agencies, etc.), academia (legal, trade and health experts from national and international universities and research bodies), and international organisations (for e.g., World Health Organisation [WHO], Council for International Organizations of Medical Sciences [CIOMS]). All the interviews were transcribed and coded for qualitative response analysis.

National interviews were conducted in New Delhi and select locations—Ahmedabad, Mumbai, Hyderabad, and Bengaluru—given the concentration of industry and pharmacy colleges in these cities. International interviews were conducted in the USA, Europe (United Kingdom,[1] Germany and Switzerland), South Africa, Singapore and Indonesia. The countries were selected based on factors including India's trading partners[2] and representations from various ongoing international cooperation initiatives—ICH, African Medicines Regulatory Harmonization (AMRH), and ASEAN.

Figure 2.1

Country-wise Break-up of Respondents

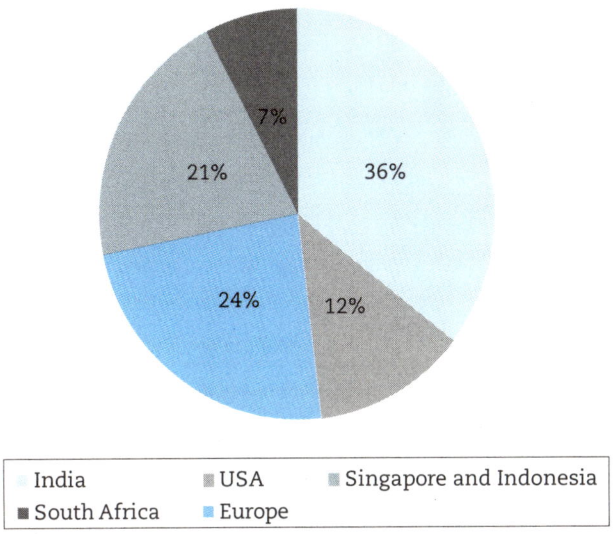

Figure 2.2

Respondents Across Stakeholder Groups

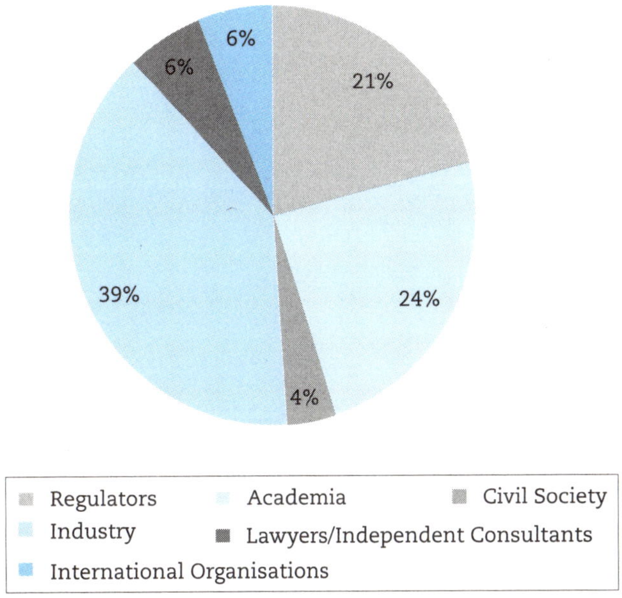

1. Our field interactions were conducted before 'Brexit'.
2. For details, please refer to Table 1 in the Appendix.

3

Analysis of Drug Registration Procedures and International Cooperation Initiatives

The present section delves into analysing the nexus between the medicine registration process and participation in international cooperation initiatives. Thus, this section provides case studies of various country contexts with diverse intrinsic characteristics, including review process of new drug applications, associated issues and their experiences in opting for different pathways of international cooperation particularly in facilitating the registration process.

3.1 India

3.1.1 Brief Background on Medicine Regulation

The regulation of pharmaceuticals in India has been a matter of concern since colonial times. In the early 20th century, India was critically dependent on imported drugs for its domestic needs and in the absence of drug regulation, there was an increased supply of spurious and adulterated drugs (Chowdhury et al. 2015). Thus regulations were initiated with the drug inquiry committee under Sir Ram Nath Chopra also known as 'Chopra Committee' which was formed due to a widespread 'gigantic quinine fraud'. The recommendations of the committee became a part of 'The Drug Bill', which was later on amended to become the Drugs and Cosmetics Act 1940 (DCA) and Drugs and Cosmetic Rules of 1945 (DCR) (Imran et al. 2013). Further, it led to the establishment of CDSCO, and the office of the Drugs Controller General (India) (DCGI).[1] As per the division of powers, CDSCO is responsible for granting approvals for clinical trials (CTs), new drugs and specialised medicinal products (vaccines, parenterals, and other high risk products) and authorisations for import and export; and State Drug Regulatory Authorities (SDRAs) are responsible for granting manufacturing, distribution and sale licences, and for inspections, sampling, testing and overall quality control of medicinal products (including investigating violations and launching prosecutions).

There are two main ministries involved in the process of drug regulation in India i.e. the Ministry of Health and Family Welfare (MoHFW) that is concerned with public health and the Ministry of Chemicals and Fertilisers which looks into promotion of the pharmaceutical industry. Additionally, there are several other ministries and acts that have a role in the medicine regulatory process.[2] A timeline of various important acts leading to the strengthening of drug regulation and attempts to align with international best practices and guidances can be seen in the Table 2 in the Appendix.

3.1.2 Medicine Registration Process (including submission and review processes, approval times, etc)

In order to register a drug in India, applicants are required to file an application for marketing authorisation to the CDSCO, and subsequently, for manufacturing licence from the SDRAs. The application is reviewed for compliance with Rule 122 and Schedule Y of the DCR. The requirements for submission of the application are based on nature and type of the drug described under the following categories:

(i) *New drugs*: The application of a new drug has to be submitted to the CDSCO and once approved by the regulator, the drug maintains the 'new drug' status for a period of four years from the date of its first approval. As per Rule 122E of DCR, a new drug is any of the following:

- One (including bulk drug substance) which has not been used in the country to any significant extent under the conditions prescribed, recommended or suggested in the labelling thereof , or/and has not been recognised as effective and safe by the licensing authority mentioned under rule 21 for the proposed claims;
- An already approved drug with modified or new claims, namely, indications, dosage, dosage form (including sustained release dosage form) and route of administration;
- A fixed dose combination of two or more drugs, individually approved earlier for

1. The CDSCO in the Directorate General of Health Services, is a division in the Ministry of Health and Family Welfare, Government of India, headed by the DCGI.

2. Other ministries are Ministry of Commerce and Industry and the Ministry of Science and Technology. Regulation of patents and; drug exports are governed by Department of Industrial Policy and Promotion and the Directorate General of Foreign Trade under the aegis of Ministry of Commerce and Industry and the Ministry of Chemical and Fertilisers respectively. Licensing and quality control and distribution maintained by CDSCO, MoHFW. The Department of Biotechnology, Ministry of Science and Technology (DST) works along with the CDSCO to frame guidelines for the regulation of biosimilars.

Figure 3.1

New Drug Registration Process at CDSCO

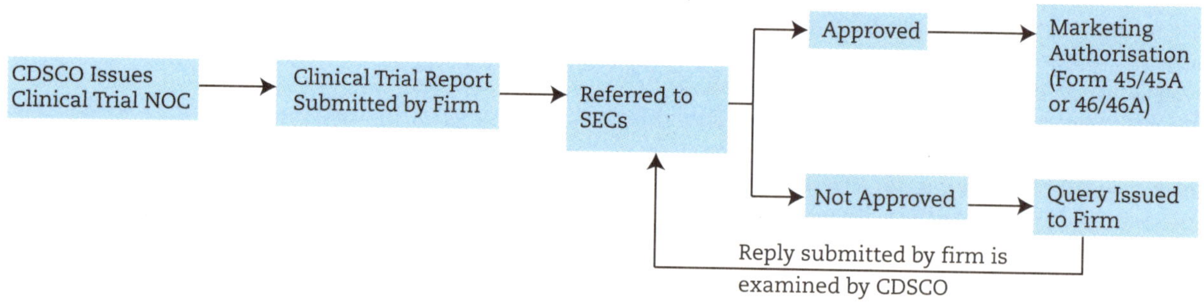

Source: Developed by Authors.

certain claims, which are now proposed to be combined for the first time in a fixed ratio, or if the ratio of ingredients in an already marketed combination is proposed to be changed, with certain claims, viz., indications, dosage, dosage form.

(ii) As per the current provisions of the DCA, after a period of four years has elapsed since its first approval, the drug ceases to be a new drug and any other manufacturer can directly apply for a manufacturing licence to the SDRA. However, with increasing public health concerns over the therapeutic equivalence of the medicines to the reference product,[3] the necessity of submission of bioequivalence (BE) data for grant of manufacturing licences have been expressed in various regulatory deliberations. In this regard, the Drugs Technical Advisory Board (DTAB)[4] has recommended that a Biopharmaceutics Classification System (BCS) should be adopted, and to begin with, BE studies be mandatory for category II and category IV of the BCS system.[5] Further, for the medicines already in the market, three years' time may be given to submit BE study data.

The process of new drug dossier review at the regulators' office (refer to Figure 3.1) starts with a pre-screening check of the application (Form 44), which is done by drug inspectors appointed as nodal officers. This pre-screening check is to ensure the completeness of the application. However, it is only an administrative check and does not provide the applicant a platform to discuss the application requirements before making the final submission to the regulator.[6] After this check, the application goes to the Subject Expert Committee (SEC), and subsequently and sequentially to the Technical Review Committee (constituted under the Directorate General of Health Services) and the apex committee. Once the application is approved by all three committees, the CDSCO issues a no objection certificate (NOC), to conduct the CT, to the applicant. The timeline prescribed by the regulator from submission of application to receiving an NOC is set 180 days for new drugs and 120 days for the application that is referred to the subsequent new drug (SND) division. However, it should be

3. As per the guidance document titled "Guidelines for Bioavailability and Bioequivalence Studies" (can be retrieved from: *http://cdsco.nic.in/html/be%20guidelines%20draft%20 ver10%20march%2016,%2005.pdf*) by CDSCO, a reference product is a pharmaceutical product that is identified by the licensing authority (CDSCO) as a 'designated reference product'—usually the global innovator's product—and contains the same active ingredient(s) as the new drug. An applicant seeking approval to market a generic equivalent must demonstrate bioequivalence with the designated reference product. For the purpose of subsequent new drug applications, the licensing authority may approve another Indian product as a designated reference product.

4. Please refer to the agenda item 4 as provided in the Minutes of 72nd DTAB meeting, accessed from *http://www.cdsco.nic.in/writereaddata/Minutes%20of%2072nd%20DTAB%20 meeting-1_07.pdf* (Last accessed on 15 April 2017).

5. According to BCS, drug substances are classified into 4 classes on the basis of the level of the aqueous permeability and solubility. Class I: High Permeability, High Solubility, Class II: High Permeability, Low Solubility, Class III: Low Permeability, High Solubility, Class IV: Low Permeability, Low Solubility. To read more, FDA Guidance on BCS can be referred from: *http://www.fda.gov/downloads/ Drugs/GuidanceComplianceRegulatoryInformation/Guidances/ ucm070246.pdf* (Last accessed on 15 April 2017).

6. As per the notice dated 28 January 2015, a provision of formal pre-submission meeting was proposed—between applicants, and CDSCO officers and subject experts—to discuss regulatory pathway in respect of specific application for approval of CT, new drug, medical device etc. However, the said proposal is yet to be formalised. See: *http://www.cdsco.nic.in/writereaddata/NOTICE15.pdf* (Last accessed on 16 January 2017).

noted that this clock would stop in case a query (or requirement additional information) has been raised by the regulator to the applicant, and the stated timeline would be reset from the date of receipt of the response.[7] After the CT report has been submitted by the applicant to the CDSCO, it is referred to the SEC. The SEC then puts up queries, if any, which are notified to the applicant by an Assistant Drug Controller at the CDCSO; otherwise DCGI on the recommendations of these various committees grants permission to market the drug as per Form 45/45A or 46/46A.[8] Note that as of now, there is no timeline proposed by the regulator for issuing grant of permission to market the new drug.

Upon analysing the new drug approvals by CDSCO from 2010-2016 (see Figure 3.2), it can be seen that over the years, the nature and type of drugs approved have changed significantly. The number of 'new drug' approvals by CDSCO in the past 6 years have declined and so has the share of fixed dose combinations in the total approved drugs.[9] The reduced new drugs applications could be attributed to the changing regulatory environment with respect to the conduct of CTs and fixed dose combinations. This may further stem from weak transmission of regulatory expectation to the applicants, possibly due to lack of clear and updated substantive procedural guidelines, along with a complex three tier review process. These issues are further elaborated in the following section.

A recent move towards improving the drug registration process promises a seamless procedure through a provision for submission of online applications through the SUGAM e-portal. SUGAM was launched, as recently as, in November 2015 and is touted to be the game changer for the regulator and the Indian pharmaceutical industry. Currently, the portal accepts applications for import and registration, medical devices and diagnostics, test, licenses, and; cosmetics, registration of ethics committees (ECs) and BA/BE studies. This is in the process of being extended to CTs, licence for pharmacy, and NOC for exports.

Figure 3.2

New Drug Approvals by CDSCO (2010-2016)

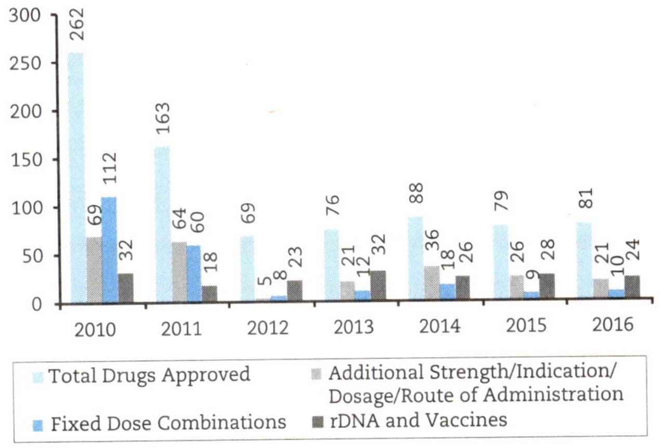

Source: Authors' compilation from list provided in CDSCO's website.

3.1.3 Issues and Concerns

During our field interactions with Indian stakeholders, much concern was expressed towards non-uniformity in the implementation of the regulatory guidelines among the SDRAs. In this regard, as a first step towards streamlining the processes, harmonisation of regulations within the country (among the SDRAs and between CDSCO and SDRAs) is widely advocated. The issue of non-uniform implementation of guidelines is further exacerbated by the lack of regulatory autonomy, as both the CDSCO and the SDRAs are umbilically tied to their parent ministries and departments of health respectively. There is also the issue regarding the lack of a comprehensive oversight over the SDRAs that would help in ensuring uniform implementation of guidelines. This affects decision-making and autonomy in a host of areas beginning with finance, recruitment and other areas of institutional policy (Chowdhury et al. 2015). These problems further accentuate the dichotomy of strong regulations and weak enforcement. Thus, there are larger systemic problems that need to be tackled for effective implementation of domestic regulations.

With regard to the registration of the medicines, the lack of procedural clarity emerged as one of the key concerns among stakeholders. This is particularly with respect to the ambiguity around the data and studies required under various application types;

7. See *http://www.cdsco.nic.in//writereaddata/upTimeline%20 CDSCO.pdf* (Last accessed on 15 April 2017).
8. Relevant forms as scheduled to DCR: Form 44: Application for grant of permission to import or manufacture a new drug or to undertake clinical trial, Form 45: Permission to import finished formulation of a new drug, Form 45 A: Permission to import raw material (new bulk drug substance), Form 46: Permission/Approval for manufacture of a new drug formulation, Form 46 A: Permission/ Approval for manufacture of raw material (new bulk drug substance).
9. The data may not be reflective of the FDCs that were given manufacturing approval by state licensing authorities—state drug regulatory authorities, prior to the approval of CDSCO. The data represents only medicine approved for human use and excludes veterinary products.

for instance, the requirement for bioequivalence studies, nature of applications which would qualify for a waiver, etc. An elaborate guidance document on the requirements for marketing authorisation of biosimilars is a welcome step in this direction.[10] However, for other areas, while regulatory guidance documents are available, the information is more on the checklist of documents than on procedural clarity. Further, complex procedures in the form of sequential involvement of various expert committees, have been flagged as a serious bottleneck resulting in unclear timelines and concerns regarding the transparency in decision-making. This has further highlighted dearth of in house capacity and high dependence on external reviewers indicating that the regulatory authority is highly understaffed for the size of the market in India. The reliance on external experts also often raises concerns over the quality of reviews, especially if the experts are engaged with other responsibilities.

Having said the above, it should also be noted that the regulator has taken towards streamlining the current processes, such as the launch of SUGAM. While SUGAM may have simplified the process for submission of applications to some extent, industry experts contend that there are still issues with its functioning such as the fact that there is no mechanism to auto forward the application to relevant departments/experts. Industry experts were of the opinion that while it is a step in the right direction, it still requires further improvements.

Most of the concerns highlighted in the preceding paragraph, came from the large players in the industry. However, the Indian pharmaceutical industry has a significant share of small and medium enterprises (SMEs)[11] which are not only engaged in production for the domestic market, but also export to countries across the world, including Nigeria, Ghana, Kenya, Russia and Sri Lanka. Some of the respondents from the SME manufacturers were apprehensive that they may be unable to bear the next wave of a stringent regulatory overhaul. This apprehension stems from their limited scale of operations. Some of our respondents reported that only about approximately 5 per cent of the SMEs register new drugs at the CDSCO.[12] This seems to suggest that a majority of these companies are engaged in the production of those formulations that are no longer classified as new drugs as per the DCA and only require the manufacturing approval of the state regulator.

3.1.4 International Cooperation

Although, India is not a party to any international initiative, it has made some efforts towards strengthening the CDSCO guidelines by refining them on the lines of international guidelines. Examples include Schedule Y of DCA.[13] Further, Schedule M of the GMP was also modified to closely align with the WHO and USFDA protocols. The CTD guidance of the ICH which has been developed for Japan,the EU, and the US has now been adopted by several other countries as well. CDSCO too, has made an attempt to adopt the CTD format for technical requirements for registration of pharmaceutical products for human use.[14,15] Additionally India has also been a part of the biannual meetings of ICH and the erstwhile global cooperation session of the ICH Steering Committee (SC) where discussions took place on a range of issues including, but not limited to, capacity-building issues and experiences/challenges in the implementation of ICH Guidelines. The most recent development on this front is India joining the ICH as an observer. During our field interactions, we learnt that the regulator's office itself has put up the proposal for its involvement at the ICH.

When the CDSCO put up the CTD guidance document for the submission of dossier, it appeared to indicate that the Indian regulator will consider taking the next step towards its electronic version i.e. the eCTD. However, this does not seem to be the case as of now. From our field interactions, it appears that SUGAM is being seen in lieu of the eCTD. The eCTD,

10. See *http://www.cdsco.nic.in/writereaddata/Bio%20Similar%20Guideline.pdf* (Last accessed on 14 April 2017).

11. Concrete numbers to gauge the network of SMEs in India is hard to find, given that a comprehensive database of manufacturers is missing. However, we do know from our field interactions that in 2007-08, there were about 10,800 SMEs in India, which subsequent to the implementation of the revised Schedule M guidelines were significantly reduced in number.

12. This is an approximate figure quoted by respondents, which we are unable to corroborate due to paucity of adequate data.

13. It defines the requirements and guidelines for import and manufacture of new drugs for sale or to undertake CTs.

14. This guidance document by CDSCO is only a draft document for feedback purposes- See *http://www.cdsco.nic.in/writereaddata/CTD%20Guidance%20Final.pdf* (Last accessed on 14 April 2017).

15. The CTD format is already in use for biological products since 2009 and this guidance document describes the format for preparation of CTD for marketing approval of pharmaceuticals for human use other than biological products (vaccines, biotechnology products, stem cell products, etc).

which is used by the industry to file applications to many countries such as the USA, the UK, Japan, Thailand, South Africa, etc., is actually quite different from what SUGAM has to offer. The eCTD has many technical complexities, being an application based process, where a document management system automatically compiles the data and submits it through a gateway to the regulator. In addition, it has provisions such as hyperlinking, xml conversions, etc. It operates like a lock and key system, where the applicant submits the application through a gateway and the regulator has a system that accepts the application in that format and aids in the process of review. Given the complexities involved in the technical requirements, it would take considerable time and resources for SUGAM to evolve on the lines of the more widely used eCTD system.

Another fairly recent development at the CDSCO, involves the establishment of a new division called the International Cell in 2014. The mandate of this cell includes review and handling of quality failure complaints of Indian made drugs, international cooperation among regulatory agencies, exchange of information regarding product recalls, etc. The cell is also involved with granting NOCs for drugs that are to be exported. Although regulating the exports from India is not explicitly the mandate of the CDSCO, it has been involved in the task owing to the increasing number of issues being flagged by international agencies.

Thus, with these efforts, India has shown the desire and ability to undergo regulatory reforms to accommodate the global industry while fostering the growth of indigenous companies and trying to avoid ethical issues. Hence, it would be interesting to examine as to how India places itself in this discourse on participating in international cooperation initiatives for registration of medicine.

3.2 United States

3.2.1 Brief Background on Medicine Regulation

Drug laws in the US have evolved over the years through a long history of trial and error. Some of the events that triggered the need for the development of stronger drug regulations world over include the Elixir Sulfanilamide incident of 1937, when over 100 people in the US died of Diethylene Glycol poisoning. Food and drug laws at that time did not require safety studies to be done for new drugs, but this incident triggered the introduction of the Federal Food, Drug and Cosmetic Act in 1938 (hereafter F, D & C Act) in the US, making it mandatory to establish the safety of a new drug prior to its marketing. Similarly, the Drug Amendments Act of 1962 (requiring stronger agency oversight over drug testing prior to market release and proof of efficacy) was enacted in the US in the aftermath of the Thalidomide disaster that took place between 1958 and 1960.[16] Such catastrophes have made the Food and Drug Administration (hereafter FDA) a very cautious regulator. This is one of the reasons behind a very gradual process of international cooperation and harmonisation that took over 20 years to evolve to its present state.

At present, the US has a centralised system of drug regulation. The FDA under the Department of Health and Human Services, regulates drugs, biologics, vaccines, cosmetics and food products as per the provisions of the F, D & C Act. The role of the states is quite limited in this respect and although a number of states have enacted 'mini' food and drug acts and statutes that prohibit healthcare and consumer fraud, but they are often not implemented since they largely duplicate the laws that FDA enforces.

3.2.2 Medicine Registration Process (including submission and review processes, approval times, etc)

Within the FDA, approval of new drugs comes under the Centre for Drug Evaluation and Research (CDER) and new biologics including vaccines, blood products, gene and tissue therapies are evaluated by the Centre for Biologics Evaluation and Research (CBER). To introduce a new product into the US market, the initial steps involve carrying out adequate pre-clinical testing, following which the originator needs to file an investigational new drug (IND) application for clinical testing on humans. There are detailed procedures for obtaining advice from FDA on the trials necessary to support a marketing authorisation application, as well as extensive written guidance concerning testing requirements. After all clinical and non-clinical testing is completed to demonstrate the safety and effectiveness of a drug, the test results are compiled into a new drug application (NDA) or biologics license application (BLA) for submission to the FDA. The actual submission of an NDA/BLA is ordinarily preceded by a pre-submission meeting to discuss the format and content of the anticipated

16. Although this sedative never received due approvals for marketing in the US, it went on sale as an over-the-counter medication in Germany in 1956 and in 46 different countries world over between 1958-1960 until its use was correlated with birth defects reported in as many as 10,000 new borns.

Figure 3.3

Review Process of NDA/BLA Application at USFDA

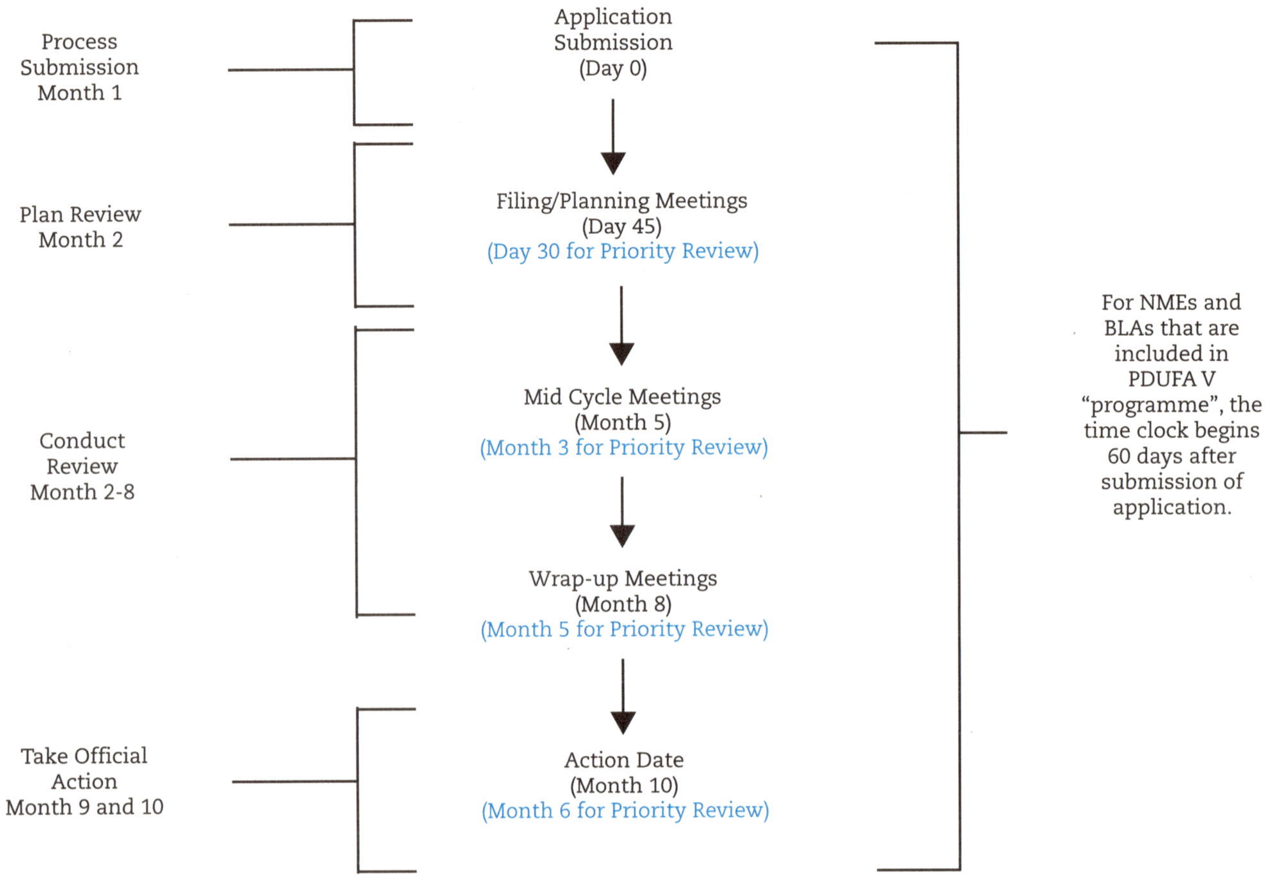

Source: Compiled by authors.

application. In cases where the application expects an expedited review, the FDA will communicate during this meeting that the review team would be targeting earlier timelines as per an expedited review.

The registration of a new product (refer to Figure 3.3) for sale in the US could be done through an NDA which further has two categories:

- Full NDA: for a NCE[17] irrespective of whether it has ever been marketed abroad or is chemically similar to some other approved drug.
- Abbreviated NDA (ANDA): for a generic version of a pioneer drug which has lost all its patents and market exclusivity.

The review time for an application depends on a number of factors. The first step for an NDA application involves determining whether it requires a 'standard' or 'priority' review. Subsequently, the review process is carried out by an interdisciplinary team under the direction of the relevant therapeutic review division within the CDER. At the end of the review cycle, the FDA issues either an approval or a complete response in case approval is denied, which informs the applicant the reasons for denial and identifies additional information required for approval.

The review time for an application depends upon the importance that it commands in meeting the public health objectives of the FDA. For an NDA application this is done by assigning each application a priority or a standard review status. A first action on a priority review application is taken within 6 months, while

17. FDA's classification of a drug as a New Molecular Entity (NME) for review purposes is distinct from FDA's determination of whether a drug product is a NCE within the meaning of the F, D & C Act. The former, in many cases, contain active moieties that have not been approved by FDA previously, either as a single ingredient drug or as part of a combination product. There are also instances where some drugs are characterised as NMEs for administrative purposes, but nonetheless contain active moieties that are closely related to active moieties in products that have previously been approved by FDA.

that on a standard review application is taken within 10 months. For ANDA applications, the public health imperative is given to a first generic i.e. the first generic versions to enter the market. Beginning 2015, the first generics applications will receive a time goal of 15 months.[18] The registration process for biologics is quite similar to that for NDA. The sponsors of biological originator products have to submit a BLA which requires almost the same information as an NDA, in the CTD format. The review of a BLA is on the same lines as that of an NDA and in order to be approved, the product must demonstrate safety, purity and potency. In 2010, a legislation was enacted for an approval process for follow-on versions of biological products, also known as biosimilars i.e. they must be highly similar to the reference product. While the legislation provides for approval of biosimilars based on analytical tests, non-clinical studies and CTs, the FDA still reserves the discretion to waive off these requirements should it feel the need to.

Figure 3.4

Number of NMEs/BLAs Fillings and Approvals at USFDA (2011-2015)

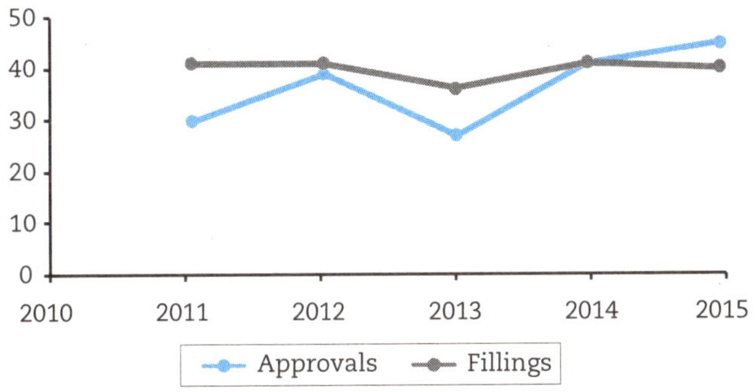

Source: Adapted from Novel Drugs 2015 Summary, USFDA.

The USFDA issues statistics on new drug approvals based on the number of orphan drugs and those first-in-class each year. Both orphan drugs and first-in-class reflect significant contribution to public health by focusing on enhancing treatment options available to the patients. To illustrate this, Figure 3.4 depicts the trend in all NDAs filed and approved between 2011 and 2015 and Figure 3.5 shows how many of the approved applications were for orphan drugs or first-in-class drugs for those years. It is interesting to note that while filings have remained fairly consistent over the years, the approval trend has not been so clear with respect to orphan drugs and first-in-class drugs. In 2015, of 45 newly approved drugs, 21 were orphan drugs and 16 were first-in-class. Both were significantly higher than the average approvals in the past 5 years (average for orphan drugs: 38% and for first-in class: 40%).

Figure 3.5

Composition of FDA New Drug Approvals

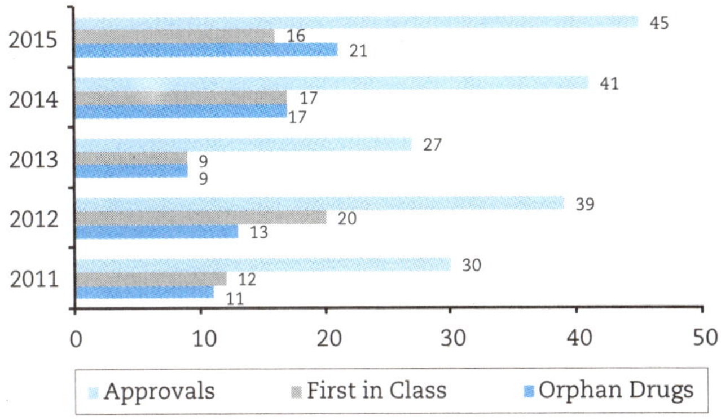

Source: Authors' compilation from various Novel New Drugs Summary Reports, USFDA.

3.2.3 Issues and Concerns

For any given company, the time that it would take to be able to launch a new product in the market plays a critical role in the company's choice of market and in certain cases may even have implications for the drug development process. Earlier, the FDA had been known to take an average of two to three years to approve a drug product after submission of the NDA, with some applications requiring much longer. After 1962, the Kefauver amendments to the F, D & C Act in the delays in drug approvals (beginning with CTs) are said to have increased to an average of 10 years (Vogel 1998). Therefore, in the 1970s and 1980s, the FDA faced criticism for the increasing drug lags as products were being approved in EU much earlier than in the US.[19] This trend changed for the first time in 1992 with the passage of the Prescription Drug User Fee Act (PDUFA). As per the provisions of the Act, the user fee to be charged from applicants were to be used to bring in a sufficient number of personnel to expedite the review process. In accordance with the PDUFA commitments, the FDA seeks to review priority applications within 8 months and standard

18. This is as per the goals set under the Generic Drug User Fee Act (GDUFA), that was brought in to expedite generic drug applications.

19. Dominguez-Urban (1997) points out that the US's relatively slower system is often defended on the grounds that it has fewer instances of market withdrawals owing to adverse reactions compared with the EU. This is because unlike US, EU chooses to bring drugs to the market relatively quickly and relies more on post-marketing surveillance to monitor drug safety.

Table 3.1

FDA's Progress Towards Meeting Backlog Goal (Cumulative Per cent of Backlog that was Issued First Action)

Submission Type	Backlogs as of October 1, 2012	FY 2013 Cumulative Percentage	FY 2013 Numbers Cleared	FY 2014 Cumulative Percentage	FY 2014 Numbers Cleared	FY 2015 Cumulative Percentage	FY 2015 Numbers Cleared
ANDA	2866	31%	888	60%	831	80%	573

Source: FY 2015 Performance Report to Congress for the Generic Drug User Fee Amendments, USFDA.

applications within 12 months, after which it issues a first response. In practice, it still can take more than a year to receive a decision on most NDA applications (Kingham and Carver 2015).[20] This is because if the FDA is unable to review the drug in the first cycle, it issues a complete response letter, and may need multiple review cycles in certain cases which could lead to an increase in the time taken to approve the drug.

In and around 2007, two particular developments with regard to generic drugs were taking place at the FDA; on the one hand there was a mounting backlog of generic drug applications at the agency which was increasing the time needed for approval tremendously, while on the other, the FDA had put across to the generic drug industry that they too should pay a user fee. This user fee, it was said, would provide the funds to garner more resources towards faster processing of applications at the agency. Thus the negotiations between the generic drug industry and the FDA for what was to be later called the Generic Drug User Fee Act (GDUFA). Subsequently, in 2012, the President of the US signed into law the Food and Drug Administration Safety and Innovation Act (FDASIA), which included authorisation for GDUFA.

Over the period of 5 years leading up to 2017 when the first cycle of GDUFA would end, the FDA put forth itself a number of performance 'time' goals for original ANDA review, amendment review, backlogs, etc. It was noted that even after GDUFA came into force, the time needed for approval[21] did not significantly go down because the agency took an initial one to two years to set up the system. So instead of a reduction in the time needed for approval, it actually went up in 2013. This was for two reasons. One, there was a greater influx of generic applications in the aftermath of GDUFA in 2012 and second, the agency began focussing on the new applications that were coming in instead of addressing the old backlog. However, they have been making gradual progress and as of FY 2015, they have been able to issue a first action[22] for 80 per cent of the backlog cases (see Table 3.1).

Other concerns identified by our respondents regarding registration also stem from lack of guidance on biosimilars and those with respect to information sharing. Another matter that has gathered attention among a number of stakeholders, is that there still remains some level of uncertainty with respect to exactly how much evidence for safety and efficacy is required and what kind of evidence would be acceptable.

3.2.4 International Cooperation

In the light of increasing domestic political pressure to expedite the drug approval process, the FDA took several measures during the early 1990s, including those of increasing cooperation with foreign regulatory agencies. Of the 24 MoUs and other cooperative agreements on pharmaceutical products that the US has signed with countries/regional groups across the world; 4 have expired and 19 are valid indefinitely, while the one with India is valid until 2019 (see table 3 in the Appendix). However, few of these cover the provisions for information exchange with respect to review documents that would aid respective regulators in the process of registration of medicines.

20. For the trend over the last nine years, see Figure 1A in the Appendix that shows the medium time to approval for all filed NDAs and BLAs under PDUFA.

21. The time to approval, however, does not necessarily imply review time. The time to approval may be significantly higher if the applications are incomplete or insufficient which leads to multiple review cycles and increase reviewer workload. For further details see *http://www.fda.gov/downloads/Drugs/DevelopmentApprovalProcess/HowDrugsareDevelopedandApproved/ApprovalApplications/AbbreviatedNewDrugApplicationANDAGenerics/UCM442070.pdf* (Last accessed on 14 April 2017).

22. The GDUFA performance goal with respect to ANDAs and its amendments, are time frames by which FDA is to take a 'first action' on an application, by wither granting an approval or a tentative approval, or if there are deficiencies that prevent approval, identifying those deficiencies to the applicant in a complete response letter or in a refusal to receive the application.

In addition, there is also limited publicly available information to evaluate accomplishments and outcomes following from these cooperative agreements (Lutter and Zorn 2016). Whether there has been any significant benefit in terms of rate of new drug introduction or any of the other outcomes remains to be seen.

One of the major developments in the last two decades, has been the setting up of the ICH, founded by the USA, Japan and the EU—much talked about as the pioneer in large scale harmonisation within the pharmaceutical sector. This initiative mainly focuses on developing quality, safety and efficacy standards for registration of pharmaceuticals that are agreed upon by all participating countries. All additional standards that have been agreed upon by the members are covered under the heading 'multidisciplinary' and include among other things, those that relate to the development of the CTD. It should be noted, however, that the CTD is nothing more than a common format and the content within this format itself is left to the discretion of individual countries.

Two formats of CTD were developed within the ICH framework; the paper based one that is known as CTD and the electronic one that is known as eCTD. While most countries even outside of the ICH have increasingly been adopting the CTD, it is the eCTD that is yet to become the norm. Even in the US, though widely used, the eCTD is not yet a legal requirement.[23] Although the FDA currently accepts eCTD applications, starting May 2017, it will make it a mandatory norm for all NDA, ANDA and BLA and from May 2018, it will be applicable for all commercial IND submissions.[24]

All the other standards developed under the ICH have been adopted by various stakeholders within the US, although without codifying these standards as rules or laws as such. The absence of new rules or laws to this effect may stem from the fact that most of these provisions are already present in the national legal framework of the US and hence obviates the need for it altogether and any minor changes or adjustments is notified through a guidance document. The agency makes its expectations quite clear in the guidance documents that it publishes and most of those in the industry understand and act accordingly when complying with various regulations and standards.

3.3 Europe

3.3.1 Brief Background on Medicine Regulation

Medicine regulation in Europe has evolved in tandem with the EU wide integration and harmonisation process, which has also played a significant role in the genesis of international initiatives like the ICH. Historically, the Thalidomide catastrophe exemplified the need for structured medicine regulations and evidence-based authorisation of medicines before their introduction into the market. Consequently, in 1965, the first pharmaceutical directive—65/65/EEC, was introduced by the council of the European Economic Community (EEC) with public health set as the cornerstone of its preamble. It laid down the provisions relating to regulation of medicinal products. It also defined baseline parameters for safety, efficacy, and quality for the purpose of evaluating a marketing authorisation application. However, there existed significant differences in the approaches to drug approval among the EU member states. In 1975, one of the first steps taken towards a joint EU position on marketing authorisations and free movement of proprietary medicines, was the formation of Committee for Proprietary Medicinal Products—CPMP (now Committee for Medicinal Products for Human Use)—a committee with experts from the competent authorities of all the member states; and establishment of a multi-state procedure for drug approval.[25] However, the role of CPMP was largely advisory and non-binding, i.e., member states were not required to follow the CPMP's recommendation (Vogel 1998: p.4). Efforts for speedier availability of medicines were reinforced with the introduction of a centralised procedure of drug approval and the subsequent formation of the European Medicines Agency (EMA), in 1995.[26] EMA

23. It should be noted that although the FDA has not amended its regulations to require the use of CTD, in practice the agency expects submission to be made in that format (Kingham and Carver 2013).

24. For further details refer to the following notice on the USFDA website *https://www.fda.gov/drugs/developmentapprovalprocess/formssubmissionrequirements/electronicsubmissions/ucm153574.htm* (Last accessed on 14 April 2017).

25. Second Council Directive of 20 May 1975, on the approximation of provisions laid down by law, regulation or administrative action relating to proprietary medicinal products. Can be accessed from: *http://eur-lex.europa.eu/legal-content/EN/TXT/PDF/?uri=CELEX:31975L0319&qid=1421942096898&from=EN* (Last accessed on 14 January 2017).

26. The EMA was actually established in 1994, however, the centralised and mutual recognition procedures did not take effect until January 1995.

is the principal agency that facilitates centralised medicine authorisation, and coordinates expertise and resources of EU member states to ensure safe, quality, efficacious medicines. Further, successive amendments supported the legal basis for medicinal products; in particular, various provisions for marketing authorisation of medicines for human use were clearly set out in the Directive 2001/83/EC and Regulation (EC) No 726/2004, and their amendments thereof. These legislations provided greater clarity on the provisions and procedures for the introduction of new medicines, including new chemical entities, generics and biosimilars in the EU market.

Common legal instruments i.e., regulations and directives—in larger scheme of affairs—have played a crucial role in shaping the harmonised pharmaceutical legislation for EU.[27] As regards to matters that are fully harmonised under EU law, there is very little divergence among the member states. There are, however, certain areas including, medicines advertising and legal status (i.e., prescription versus over the counter) of drugs not authorised in the centralised procedure that are only partially harmonised, for which there remains significant differences in national requirements. Further, there are areas which are not harmonised at all and hence there exist differences among the member states, these include provision of healthcare, payer structures—pricing and reimbursement of medicines.

3.3.2 *Medicine Registration Process (including submission and review processes, approval times, etc)*

In order to introduce a medicinal product in EU (or specific member state(s)), the first essential step is to obtain marketing authorisation from the competent authority (ies). There are various routes for registering a medicine in Europe, depending upon the nature and the type of medicine. During our field interactions, we learnt that clarity in regulatory procedures of medicines registration is one of the most consequential factors for a company to introduce the medicine in a country. Europe stands out as an interesting case study of harmonisation of marketing authorisation procedures, which has significantly contributed to streamlining the drug approval process. To apply for a marketing authorisation in the EU, the applicant must be established within the European Economic Area.

Table 3.2

Legal Basis for Applications for Marketing Authorisation in Europe

Type of Application	*Article under Directive 2001/83/EC*
Full application	Article 8(3)
Well-established use application	Article 10a
Fixed dose combination application	Article 10b
Informed consent application	Article 10c
Generic application	Article 10(1)
Hybrid application	Article 10(3)
Similar biological application	Article 10(4)

Source: Compiled by the authors from information provided in EMA's website.

There are four different routes to apply for a marketing authorisation in EU—national procedure, centralised procedure, decentralised procedure and mutual recognition procedure (as explained below, also please see flowchart—Figure 3.6—for further procedural clarity). The applicants for marketing authorisations are required to communicate the intent to submit the applications well in advance of the anticipated date of submission, and also request for a pre-submission meeting with the regulator. As both the EMA and the competent authorities of member states have a heavy workload, these interactions help bringing in clarity regarding regulatory requirements and improve quality of submissions, which further facilitates the maintenance of timelines. The applicants are required to submit sufficient and consistent data to demonstrate quality, safety, and efficacy of the products with the dossiers to be submitted in eCTD format. The requirements and legal basis for marketing authorisation applications have been laid in the articles as described in Table 3.2. In addition to general guidelines on requirements for approval, there are procedures at the national and EU level for applicants to obtain advice on testing requirements for specific drugs. The procedures vary at the national level, but in most cases include opportunities for in-person meetings as well as written responses to questions. At the EU level, there is a Scientific Advice Working Party of the Committee for Medicinal Products for Human Use (CHMP), which provides written advice on such matters.

27. While a regulation is binding on all the member states in its entirety, a Directive is mainly a direction for EU member states to achieve a certain goal—member states have to adopt measures to transpose the directive into their national laws, within a stipulated deadline. Further, for regulatory clarity among the stakeholders—in case of pharmaceuticals—there are guidelines that are non-binding in nature, however, represent a harmonised EU position in the concerned subject.

Figure 3.6
Different Regulatory Pathways of Obtaining Marketing Authorisation in Europe

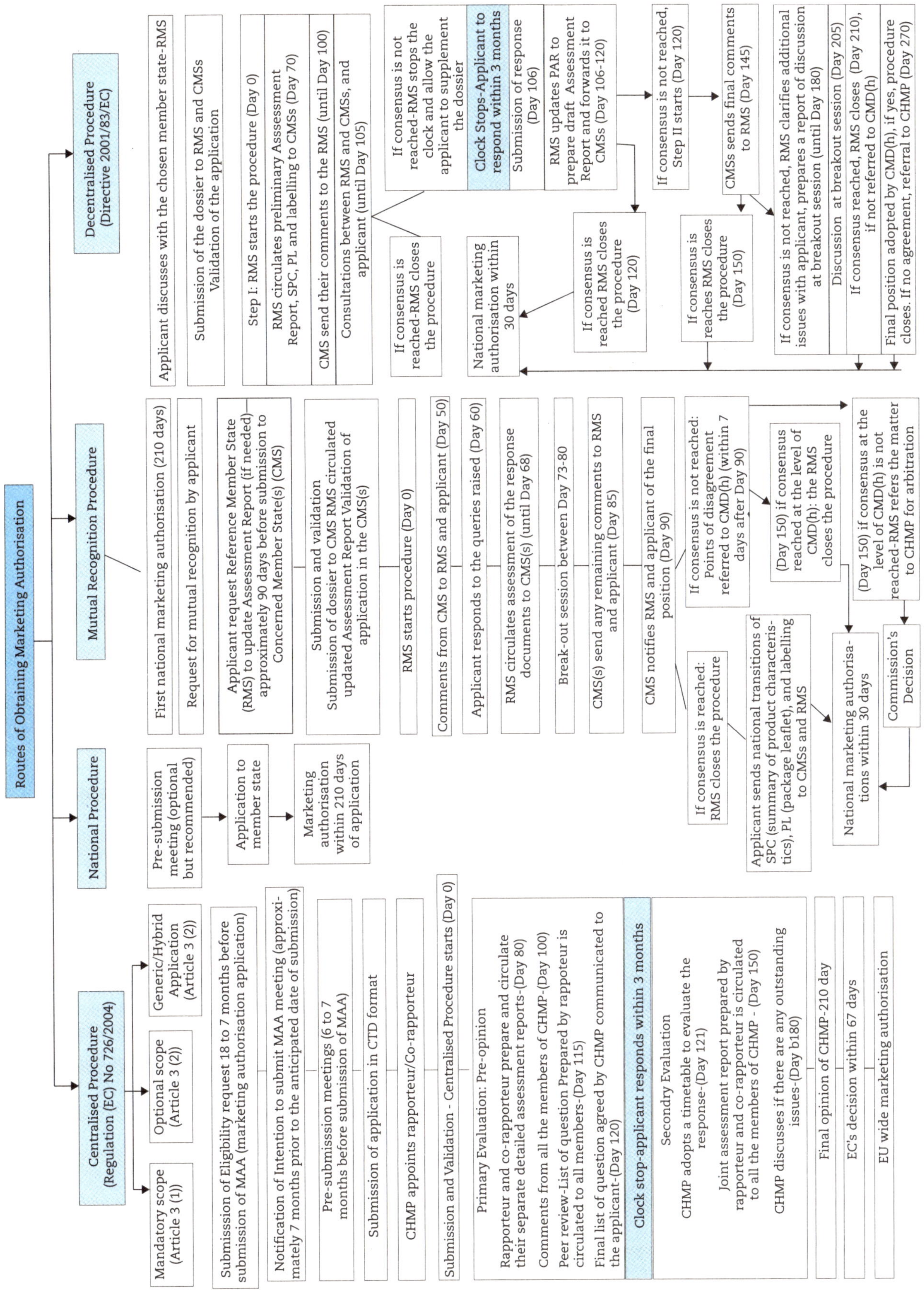

(i) Certain specified products,[28] fall under the mandatory scope of union or centralised procedure and such an application must be made directly to the EMA. Additionally, generic[29] versions of the products approved under centralised procedure may also apply for marketing authorisation under centralised procedure. CHMP carries out the scientific evaluation of the applications and sends its scientific opinion to the European Commission (EC). CHMP adopts its opinion on or before the 210th day,[30] after which the EC drafts the decision and, in consultation with the member states, through the relevant standing committee, adopts the decision and grants a European marketing authorisation which is binding on all member states.[31] The review timelines of 210 regulatory days (excluding the time taken by the applicant to respond to queries raised by EMA) are statutory and are, reportedly, strictly adhered to by the EMA.

Interestingly, in the harmonised framework of the EU, there is no provision for parallel evaluations of national marketing authorisation applications by member states. In case, the product does not fall under the scope of the centralised procedure, an applicant can opt for national procedure (in case of introducing a medicine in only one member state) or mutual recognition procedure or decentralised procedure (in case of introducing medicine in multiple member states). These procedures are primary authorisation pathways to introduce a generic into the EU market.

(ii) National marketing authorisations[32] are meant for the applicants who wish to market their medicinal product in only one member state. Under this procedure, marketing authorisation is granted by the competent authorities of the member state. For instance, Bundesinstitut für Arzneimittel und Medizinprodukte (BfArM) is responsible for granting marketing authorisations for medicinal products(other than biologics) that are marketed only in Germany.

(iii) Under the mutual recognition procedure,[33] if a product is lawfully sold in one member state of the EU, then it can be sold in another member state, unless there are serious concerns related to public safety, health, or the environment in that member state. Under the said procedure, the national authorisation granted by one member state (the reference member state[RMS])[34] has to be recognised by the competent authorities of the other member states (the concerned member states [CMS]). Any national marketing authorisation granted by a member state can be used to support an application for its mutual recognition by other member states.

28. Medicinal products, authorised under Regulation (EC) No 726/2004, containing new active substances which constitute a significant therapeutic, derived from biotechnology, for orphan medicinal products, for medicinal products for human use which contain an active substance authorised in the European Community after 20 May 2004 and which are intended for the treatment of AIDS, cancer, neurodegenerative disorders or diabetes. Also, as per Article 3(2) of Regulation (EC) No 726/2004, defines the 'optional scope' of the centralised procedure, whereby, the applicant may apply for union or centralised marketing authorisation, upon demonstrating that the medicinal product constitutes a significant therapeutic, scientific or technical innovation which is in the interest of patients and public health at large.

29. The applicant of generic medicines can submit abridged dossier (not requiring results of pre-clinical tests and clinical trials) demonstrating that the medicinal product is a generic of a reference medicinal product upon expiration of the 8 year exclusivity period (regulatory incentives). Regulatory data incentives includes regulatory exclusivity (8 years), market data exclusivity (2 years) provisions for a new drug, and one additional year in case of significant therapeutic advancement is approved in first 8 years of data exclusivity. The authorised generic product can only be launched in the market after the expiry of market protection, i.e., until 10 years have elapsed from the authorisation of the reference product.

30. The opinion of CHMP (positive or negative), is subject to appeal. And from opinion to decision, the overall duration should be within 67 days.

31. A new national marketing authorisation for the same medicinal product would be issued only in case the therapeutic indications are different in national and central marketing authorisations.

32. National marketing authorisations initially lasts five years and is usually subject to one renewal.

33. Since 1 January 1998, the mutual recognition procedure is compulsory for all medicinal products to be marketed in a member state other than that in which they were first authorised. The legal provisions for mutual recognition procedure and decentralised procedure are underlined in the Directive 2001/83/EC and Regulation (EC) No 764/2008. Evaluation procedure undertaken by the member state may take up to 210 days (which excludes the time taken to provide further information).

34. The selection of the RMS is at the discretion of the applicant, based on many factors including preference for local regulator, therapeutic expertise of the competent authority, size of the market, response of the regulator while discussing application, etc. Raymond and Humphreys (2013) assert that the distribution of RMS is skewed with only five national competent authorities (Denmark, UK, Germany, Netherlands, and Sweden) evaluating greater than 80 per cent of the applications received.

(iv) In the decentralised procedure, identical applications can be submitted simultaneously to the competent authorities of RMS and CMS(s). The applicant discusses the proposed submission of date with the selected RMS, after which the application is submitted to RMS and the notified CMSs for validation. Since the procedure starts only upon validation from the CMSs, the time taken for validation can extend the timelines in case there are country-specific requirements (EGA Regulatory Efficiency Report 2015: 28). After repeated consultations among RMS, CMSs and the applicant, a draft assessment report is prepared by the RMS. In case a consensus is reached between RMS and CMSs, the RMS closes the procedure and the respective CMSs grants national marketing authorisation.

In the case of both mutual recognition procedure and decentralised procedure, if the member states are unable to reach a consensus, then it has to be notified to the Coordination Group for Mutual Recognition and Decentralised Procedures for Human Medicinal Products (CMD(h)). In case CMD(h) is unable to resolve the issue, it goes for arbitration at the CHMP. Upon the completion of the procedures, national marketing authorisation is granted by each CMS.

The only difference between the decentralised procedure and mutual recognition procedure is that in case of mutual recognition, one of the member states has already granted a national marketing authorisation, which then is mutually recognised by CMS. The decentralised procedure is applicable to medicinal products that have not received a market authorisation at the time of the application—it is a first time application.

While mutual recognition involves tight timetables that are difficult to meet in case there are disparities among the CMS with the assessment report of RMS. A predominant view from the field interactions was that, over the years, decentralised procedure as an improved successor to mutual recognition procedure, gained popularity over mutual recognition procedure (also see Figure 3.7). In the decentralised procedure, an applicant can not only apply in multiple member states simultaneously, but also has the opportunity of iterative regulatory advice from the RMS before getting into the full regulatory application process. The decentralised procedure provides various opportunities for building consensus before the final approval (Raymond and Humphreys 2013: 391).

Figure 3.7

Data Representing Finalised Procedures of Mutual Recognition Procedure and Decentralised Procedure for the Period 2006-2015

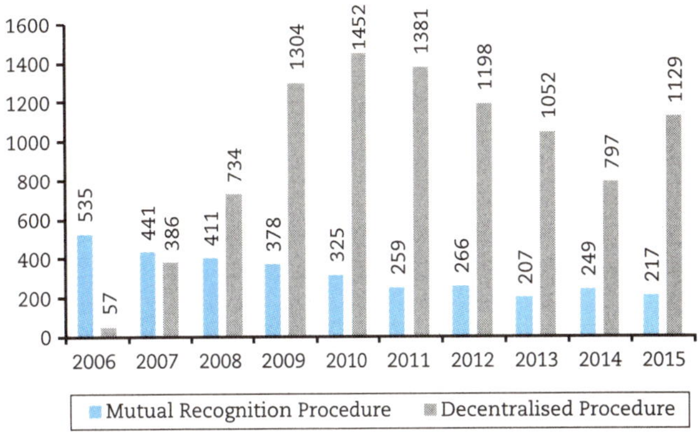

Source: Compiled by the authors from Annual Coordination Group for Mutual Recognition and Decentralised Procedures-Human (CMDh) Statistics.

Figure 3.8

Positive Opinion by CHMP for Applications under Centralised Procedure

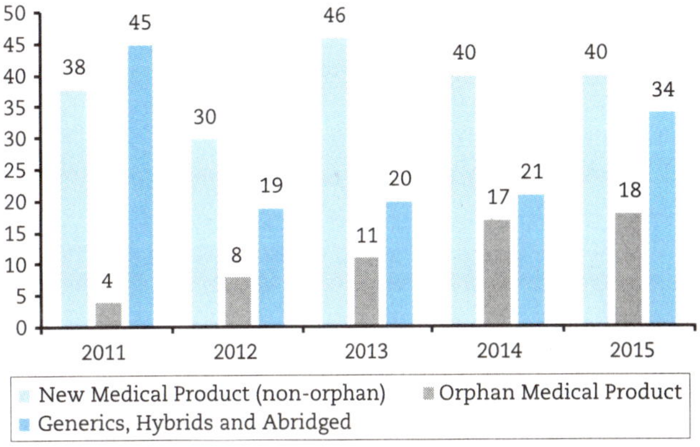

Source: Authors' compilation from *Annual Report EMA, 2015*.

As far as promotion of public health is concerned, in cases where the medicine fulfils an unmet medical need or public health emergency is crucial from the point of view of therapeutic innovation, EMA offers Facilitated Regulatory Pathways (FRPs)[35] including 'accelerated assessment,'[36] conditional approvals, and schemes like PRIME (PRIority MEdicines). Out of 41 new active substances approved by EMA, 32 per cent of the products benefitted from at least one FRP in 2015 (R&D Briefings 59, CIRS). Increased focus on

35. FRPs are referred to as alternatives to standard regulatory pathways that can accelerate the development, submission, regulatory review and patient access to important medicines with a positive benefit-risk balance for serious diseases or unmet medical need.

36. The expedited timeline is of 150 days.

public health is also reflected in, as shown in Figure 3.8, increased positive opinions on orphan medicinal products over the period of 2011 to 2015.

Lastly, the final launch of the new medicine depends upon the time taken by the pricing and reimbursement mechanism, which is still a national mandate and differs from one member state to another.

3.3.3 *Issues and Concerns*

Successful implementation of various EU procedures varied among the member states based upon their competencies. For instance, the principle of mutual recognition is contingent upon an array of factors including, the level of trust in the decision-making of a regulator, given the differing level of resources with the competent authorities across the member states, stringency of timelines, and the sovereignty of individual member states to decide upon the need and the relevance of the medicines to be introduced to their population. One of the major views that were expressed in our field interactions highlighted, in early years of its introduction, mutual recognition did not garner immediate acceptance among the competent authorities of the member states as a procedure to grant marketing authorisation of pharmaceutical products, and was seen as a serious risk to the public health goal. Despite clear harmonised rules, concerns arose because of lack of trust in decision-making and assessments of other agencies. However, with the increased regulatory consultations among the member states and endorsement by the heads of agencies, mutual recognition procedure did gain popularity and succeeded in facilitating timely introduction of medicines in Europe. Also, the best practice guide by the European Federation of Pharmaceutical Industries' Association and meetings of Mutual Recognition Facilitation Group (MRFG) (now CMD(h)) helped to improve time both for initiating a mutual recognition procedure and the granting of national marketing authorisations.[37]

Further, the harmonised procedures benefitted the differences in the review practices that surfaced with the expansion of EU membership in 2004. This is because, traditionally, the Eastern European countries reportedly had different review proceedings. As shown in Figure 3.9, disagreements among member states have declined over the years, which, inter alia, could be attributed to the introduction of more systematic decentralised procedure (DCP). Work sharing and multinational review teams have also been useful in reducing differences and, developing expertise and capacity in the member states.

As regards to adherence to the review timelines, EMA and competent authorities of most member states have project managers, in addition to scientific experts, to ensure that the procedural timelines are met. However, the timelines are often affected by factors which are beyond the control of project managers such as, validation period by CMS, time taken to resume clock stop after the response for queries is received from the applicant, and time taken in granting of national marketing authorisation, etc.

Figure 3.9

Finalised Mutual Recognition Procedures versus Referrals to CMDh

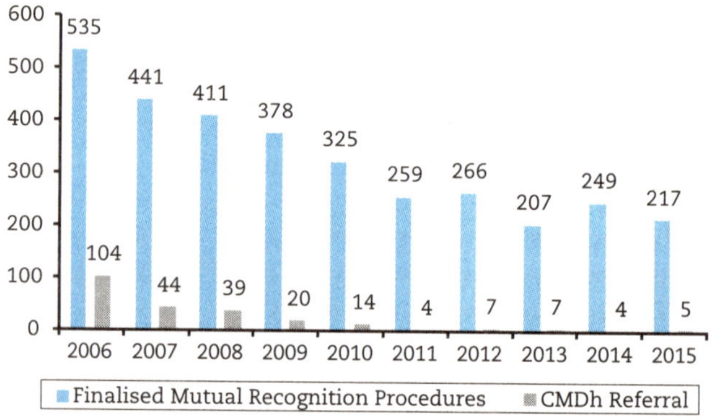

Source: Compiled from Annual Coordination Group for Mutual Recognition and Decentralised Procedures-Human (CMDh) Statistics.

3.3.4 *International Cooperation*

As discussed before, the globalisation of the pharmaceutical industry and increased regulatory scope has provided an impetus to international cooperation in various aspects of medicine regulation. Europe is considered to be one of the most successful cases for internal harmonisation in various sectors and it is believed that it has worked well because it was embedded in a larger scheme of affairs—the principle of free movement of goods within the EU. As differences in national technical requirements continue to exist, the principle of mutual recognition has further facilitated faster access to a single market, to the products which are not subject to EU harmonisation.

37. See: Extract from the *Third General Report on the Activities of the European Agency, for the Evaluation of Medicinal Products 1997*, retrieved from: *http://www.hma.eu/fileadmin/dateien/Human_Medicines/CMD_h_/Statistics/1997_mrr_statistics.pdf* (Last accessed on 9 January 2017).

The process of internal harmonisation has facilitated the streamlining of medicine registration in the EU, however, its effective implementation took several years. At present, the submission of marketing authorisation application is greatly facilitated by the various procedures discussed above, also mutual recognition of the reference assessment has provided for pooling of regulatory resources.

Internationally, in the realm of medicine regulations, EC is one of the founding members of ICH, and works with other international organisations and standardisation initiatives along with EMA, namely, International Coalition of Medicines Regulatory Authorities (ICMRA); Pharmaceutical Inspections Co-operation Scheme (PIC/S). EMA also has bilateral agreements with the regulators of the USA, Canada, Japan, Switzerland, Australia, New Zealand, and Israel. Further, it supports the ECs collaboration on pharmaceuticals with China, India, and Russia.[38] The process of harmonisation[39] in Europe, although largely trade driven, has tremendously benefitted the medicines regulations. Even the ICH process was prompted by the need to have common standards in order to facilitate trade between the participating countries. The harmonised ICH guidelines have immensely contributed to streamlining the regulations, particularly with respect to having agreed upon a common submission format—CTD.

With specific reference to the registration of medicines, the EU has adopted ICH CTD (and now eCTD) which is of special relevance for the companies applying in multiple jurisdictions (in addition to the EU). Even for SMEs, CTD has provided a framework to operate and enhance access to different markets, as it brings about clarity in the format of dossiers. While the benefits of CTD have contributed to bringing about a more efficient process of application submission, the field interactions suggested that the evidence on its direct role in reducing the approval times is limited.

Additionally, EMA initiates various efforts in the direction of facilitating registration of medicines outside the EU in the form of provisions under Article 58 procedure, and real time sharing of assessment reports of generic products, with non-EU regulators in IGDRP. In the context of cooperation with the WHO and collaboration with the EC and Bill and Melinda Gates Foundation, Article 58 of Regulation (EC) No 726/2004 enables the EMA to provide support for capacity building in Low and Middle Income Countries (LMICs) by providing scientific assistance to non-EU member countries for the evaluation of certain medicinal products for human use that are intended exclusively for markets outside of the EU. This facilitates rapid access to important new medicinal products, for people living outside the EU, targeting diseases including HIV/AIDS, malaria, TB, etc.

3.4 ASEAN

3.4.1 *Drug Registration Procedures and International Cooperation*

The development of the ASEAN[40] region was largely trade driven with the focus on achieving economic integration in Southeast Asia. Efforts have been made since then to build harmonisation of standards and bring about regulatory convergence, taking into account the diversities that exist in its member states (Pettman 2013). For pharmaceuticals, steps to achieve harmonisation were initiated through the ASEAN Consultative Committee for Standards and Quality (ACCSQ) which was formed by the ASEAN Economic Ministers in 1992. It was aimed at facilitating and complementing the objectives of the ASEAN Free Trade Area (AFTA)[41] and to eventually implement the MRAs (Ratanawijitrasin 2007). This led to pharmaceutical harmonisation initiative that facilitated the objective of AFTA by enforcing cooperation in the field of public health through the establishment of Pharmaceuticals Product Working Group (PPWG) in 1999.

The PPWG reviewed the existing pharmaceutical requirements of its member countries as well as other international standards such as the ICH and WHO. New guidelines were developed in areas where guidelines were not present or were not applicable

38. As per the information available at *http://www.ema.europa.eu/ema/index.jsp?curl=pages/partners_and_networks/general/general_content_000214.jsp&mid=WC0b01ac058003176d* (Last accessed on 15 September 2016).

39. Europe is harmonised by European Directives, which individual member State governments have to enforce within their own jurisdiction, that include detailed guidance on all the procedures required to authorised drugs and the requirements thereof.

40. ASEAN was established on 8 August 1967 in Bangkok by the five original member countries: Indonesia, Malaysia, the Philippines, Singapore, and Thailand. Brunei Darussalam joined on 8 January 1984, Vietnam on 18 July 1995, Laos and Myanmar on 23 July 1997, and Cambodia on 30 April 1999.

41. AFTA is a collective effort to reduce/eliminate tariffs in intra-ASEAN trade in the goods sector.

to ASEAN members (Lakkis 2008). Although ASEAN accepted several guidelines of the ICH but it did review the suitability of these to its own region. A relevant example can be of the climate stability conditions as ICH zone IV requirements were not suitable for ASEAN. Consequently, ASEAN raised this issue and WHO sub divided it into additional stability conditions called Zone IV B, for hot and humid climate conditions. It was adopted by many non-ASEAN countries as well (Lakkis 2008 and Speers et al. 2016).

Some of the key documents produced by this group include the ASEAN Common Technical Requirements (ACTR) and the ASEAN Common Technical Document (ACTD) for pharmaceutical product registration for human use. The ACTD provides an outline of administrative data, quality and safety—which are common to all ASEAN members and the ACTR contains guidelines on quality, safety, and efficacy which help in the preparation of application dossiers so that they are consistent with the requirements of all ASEAN Drug Regulatory Authorities (Pettman 2013). The ACTD is very similar to, although slightly less extensive than, the ICH CTD. Another distinction between ICH CTD and ACTD is the focus of the latter on the registration of generic products, due to the predominance of the generic industry in the region. Although preparing ACTD in addition to ICH CTD is cumbersome for the industry[42] but it does help as one dossier i.e. the ACTD can be submitted to all ASEAN countries together (Lakkis 2008). Nonetheless, country specific requirements still exist among the member countries, and many authorities[43] still require new registrations in their own regional documents along with elements of ACTD which is a matter of concern for companies (Speers et al. 2016).

The new harmonised system of application using ACTD and ACTR has been made effective since 2004, however owing to the need for countries to amend their national laws, they were given flexible timelines.[44] Online submission portals[45] are used in some states but there is no centralised route for simultaneous submission across ASEAN (Speers et al. 2016).

Among ASEAN member states, even though the submission format is harmonised, the review is still the mandate of each country's regulatory authority. Due to poor infrastructure and limited human resources in most of the countries in the region, the review of applications is dependent on the provision of the Certificate of Pharmaceutical Product (CPP) issued by a reference or an advanced country (Wong 2003). But even then, the review timelines are long which leads to an approval lag in the countries. Submission lag[46] is another concern which has a huge impact on the introduction of medicine in some countries (Liberti et al. 2012). A recent study (*Center of Medicine Research International Report*, 2001 as cited in Wong 2003) showed that companies would prefer to submit their registration dossier simultaneously in Asia when they submit the NDA to developed countries but are unable to do so and hence the lag. ASEAN PPWG and ACTD were also developed to ease this procedure and reduce the timelines to approval in this region. It was pointed out by the field respondents that a company would first submit the dossier in countries which accept the ICH CTD as a number of countries would be covered in one go. Subsequently, it would move on to the ASEAN region using the common ACTD format and then focus on other countries that use their local formats. Hence ACTD was expected to bring the drug earlier to the market but no such reduction in submission lag has been reported.

Concerns have been raised to focus on joint assessments—which will enable the less-experienced regulatory authorities to learn from the competent experts at more experienced authorities such as Health Sciences Authority (HSA)—Singapore's national drug regulatory body. Consequently, discussions at the ASEAN level led to the establishment of a programme called 'Supporting the Implementation of ASEAN Harmonized Requirements for Drug Registration' (SIAHR) with the WHO, but it is still at a preliminary phase.[47] Regional industry associations at ASEAN—called the ASEAN Pharmaceutical Club (APC), composed of members from the local generic industry and

42. This primarily holds for cases where the applicant is catering to both ICH and ASEAN region.

43. For instance, in Laos, submission requires the safety and efficacy documents outlined in parts I-IV of the ACTD and the specific 'LP2' form.

44. The trial period for ACTD began in 2003 while its complete implementation was postponed until 2009. Singapore and Malaysia adopted it by 2005, Thailand by 2006, Indonesia and Vietnam by 2007 and other countries followed.

45. Such as PRISM (Pharmaceutical Regulatory Information System) in Singapore and Quest in Malaysia.

46. Submission lag is referred to as the time from which a product has been granted market authorisation in its first market to the time that its application is submitted for review by an authority in emerging markets.

47. See *http://apac-asia.com/images/achievements/pdf/5th/ATIM_06_Dato'AISAH.pdf* (Last accessed on 7 April 2017).

the ASEAN Pharmaceutical Research Industry Associations (APRIA), comprising of representatives of multinational companies—are a part of the ASEAN meetings and have supported such concerns at the forum.

MRAs have been another initiative under the harmonisation scheme of ASEAN. PPWG identified that it is possible only after ACTR and ACTD is fully implemented. The identified areas in which discussion was initiated are Good Manufacturing Practices (GMP) inspections and bioavailability and bioequivalence (BABE) studies. Although MRA on BABE studies is yet to be implemented, MRA on GMP is in progress and has been achieved by some member states.[48] Countries that have not been able to implement it are encouraged to accept the reports of other members. The reason that the impact of MRA on GMP is not uniform throughout the region is the lack of trust among countries, which makes cooperation difficult. In certain cases, developed countries find it difficult to trust developing countries with their decisions; a concern that was observed in our field interactions as well. This is one of the key debates surrounding MRAs; as though they help in enhancing the flow of goods between countries yet they are unable to be aligned with the principles of a single market. Hence, it often leads to bilateral agreements, as the more developed countries in the group take the lead. This gives rise to the possibility of a two-stage harmonisation process where the more developed ASEAN economies enter into MRAs with other developed ASEAN economies due to compatibility between their regulatory regimes (Pettman 2013).

The countries in ASEAN are at different stages of development in terms of their level of growth, infrastructure available to the health regulatory authority, health expenditure, regulations related to quality and safety of drugs, etc. Among the members, most are low income countries except for Singapore and Malaysia (Venkateswarlu et al. 2014). Therefore, the willingness and participation of these countries in the harmonisation initiative also varies, thus affecting the level of implementation. Nevertheless, a regional cooperation initiative is often considered better and more feasible than a global one, as similar countries find it easy to trust and collaborate with each other. Such interactions among regional initiatives will help in further collaboration.

To sum up, harmonisation in the drug registration process in ASEAN has been a gradual process with the degree of success varying among members. This is due to differences in the background of the country, level of economic development, presence of local industry, willingness to harmonise, and regulatory requirements and capacities. The cooperation in the registration process has been complicated to some extent as each country has a separate review process and certain country specific requirements. The problem arises due to different objectives and interpretations of varied governments. Though ASEAN works on the principle of mutual consensus, yet implementation has been weak even after the decision is made. Hence, it is suggested that the key is to invest more capital and resources in the harmonisation process. In addition to this, it is important that the more developed states help and train the less developed ones and work jointly with them to achieve uniform implementation of guidelines (Pettman 2013). This will speed up the launch of drugs and improve access to medicine.[49] Thus, there is a need to work on minimising the divergences that exist among the member states so that ASEAN becomes a model for regional cooperation.

Two of the ASEAN member states—Singapore and Indonesia—have been taken as case studies owing to their varied country characteristics and experience in relation to international cooperation.

3.4.2 Singapore

3.4.2.1 Brief Background on Medicine Regulation

Singapore is one of the most developed economies with a population of about 5.6 million[50] and a per capita health expenditure as high as USD 2,752[51] in 2014. The development of the pharmaceutical industry in Singapore is mainly due to its strong infrastructure and science-based regulation, which has made it a manufacturing centre for biomedical products. In June 2000, Singapore had declared its intention to become the biomedical hub of Asia and since then, there has been remarkable progress in the field. The ecosystem in the country along with

48. Singapore, Indonesia, Malaysia and Thailand are a part of PIC/s and have implemented MRA on GMP.

49. *https://www.adb.org/publications/better-regulation-medicines-stronger-regional-health-security* (Last accessed on 7 April 2017).

50. See *http://www.who.int/countries/sgp/en/* (Last accessed on 7 April 2017).

51. See *http://data.worldbank.org/indicator/SH.XPD.PCAP?contextual=aggregate&end=2014&locations=SG&start=1995&view=chart* (Last accessed on 7 April 2017).

a sound regulatory framework has led to early drug discovery, helped in ensuring patient safety and enabled early phase CTs. In addition to this, the country offers business incentives and a protective regulatory environment with strong intellectual property laws to ensure equal treatment of local and foreign companies, making it a standard model of a successful free market economy (Lakkis 2010 and Lee 2015).

One of the key milestones in the history of health products regulation in Singapore is the enactment of Medicines Act, 1975. It provided a comprehensive framework for the regulation of medicinal products, licensing of medicinal product importers, manufacturers, assemblers, wholesale and dealers, registration of premises and regulation of medical advertisements and promotion. The provisions of the Act were implemented by the Drug Administration Division of the Ministry's Pharmaceutical Department, but in phases so that stakeholders had sufficient time to meet the new requirements. Henceforth in 1999, with the expansion of its regulatory functions and responsibilities, this department was renamed the National Pharmaceutical Administration (NPA). In 2001, NPA was consolidated with four former national agencies,[52] which led to the establishment of the Health Science Authority (HSA), Singapore's current health regulatory body. After a few organisational changes within the HSA, the Health Products Regulation Group (HPRG) was formed in 2007 (Lee 2015). In Singapore, pharmaceuticals were regulated by two acts namely, the Medicines Act (as discussed above) and the Health Products Act (HPA),[53] 2007 (Lakkis 2010). But with a recent change in legislation, HSA has streamlined and transferred the existing regulatory controls for pharmaceutical products by merging both, the Medicines Act and the Poisons Act, into a single legislation, i.e., the HPA, with effect from 1 November 2016. Under the HPA, pharmaceutical products, or conventional chemical and biologic drugs, are referred to as TP (therapeutic products), and regulatory controls are stratified based on the risk profiles of the products.[54]

52. Namely, Centre for Drug Evaluation, Institute of Science and Forensic Medicine, Product Regulation Department and Singapore Blood Transfusion Service.

53. The Health Products Act was enacted to expand regulatory practice to include health products, such as medical devices, cosmetics, traditional Chinese medicines and health supplements.

54. See *http://www.hsa.gov.sg/content/hsa/en/News_Events/HSA_Updates/2016/tpportoverhealthproductsact.html* (Last accessed on 10 April 2017).

3.4.2.2 Medicine Registration Process (Including Submission and Review Processes, Approval Times, etc)

Singapore is an attraction for multinational pharmaceuticals companies as the regulatory procedures are well defined, efficient and timely. HSA offers a comprehensive registration procedure beginning with the pre-submission preparation (an enquiry or a meeting) which is one of the most important steps. The enquiry helps in choosing the evaluation route and arranging a pre submission consultation meeting with the HSA if there is a need. There are 2 product types, namely, a NDA and a generic drug application (GDA) and three major evaluation routes that offer flexibility to the applicants of selecting the route that best meets their needs. The three routes are discussed below (Guidance on Medicinal Product Registration in Singapore, 2011).

i. Full review: Applies to any product that has not been approved by any DRA at the time of submission. The applicant may request a priority review for a life-saving drug if it claims to cater to unmet medical needs.

ii. Abridged review: Applies to any product that has been evaluated and approved by at least one DRA.

iii. Verification review: Applies to any product that has been evaluated and approved by HSA's reference DRAs, which include the EMA,[55] the USFDA, Health Canada, TGA and UK MHRA.[56]

For faster introduction of generics in Singapore, the country has given a separate registration procedure for India under Comprehensive Economic Cooperation Agreement (CECA). Given that India is one of the biggest producers of generic medicines, this was introduced for the registration of the products manufactured in India and to facilitate their quicker market authorisation in Singapore. The timeline is shorter for such products (90 days rather than 120 days) through the verification review route which is expected to speed up the registration process.

Application submission comprises two of parts: the PRISM (Pharmaceutical Regulatory Information System) application form and the registration dossier.

55. For products approved via the centralised procedure.

56. For products approved via the national procedure or where MHRA acted as the RMS for the MRP or decentralised procedures in Europe.

Figure 3.10

Drug Registration Process in Singapore

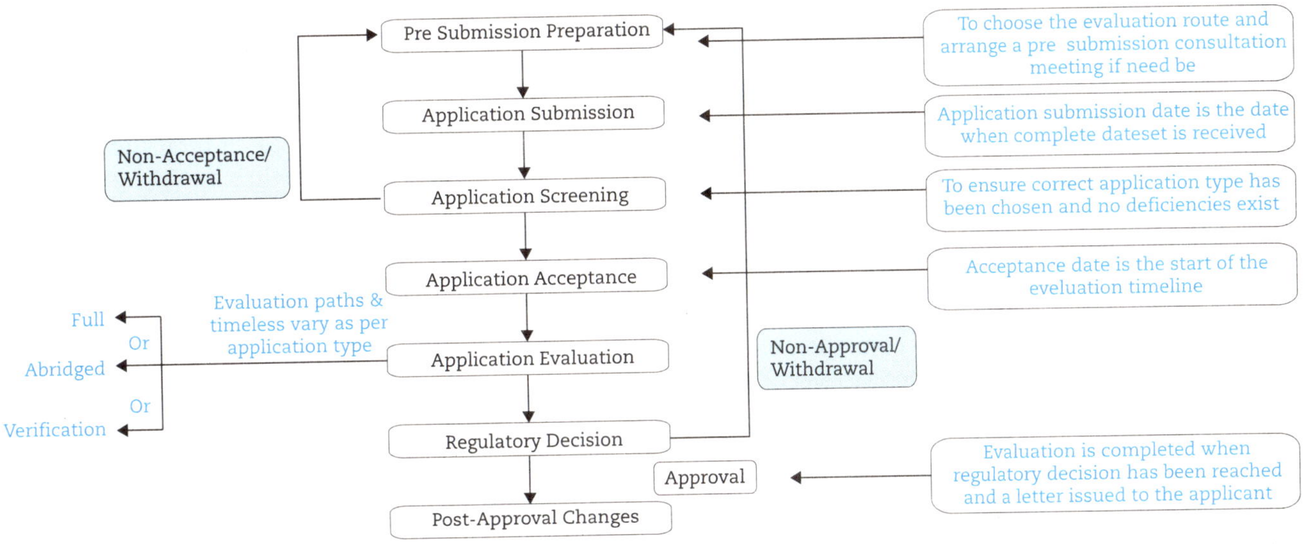

Source: Compiled by authors.

All applications must be made on-line via the PRISM portal. Singapore allows the registration dossier to be in either ICH CTD or ACTD format. Due to the wider acceptance of ICH CTD, a need has been felt to encourage its adoption on a wider scale but due to the effort and time spent in adoption of ACTD[57], ASEAN countries are not very willing to do away with it. In order to move towards a greener environment, submission of the complete registration dossier has been made electronic with the exception of documents that require proof of authenticity.[58] eCTD, as mentioned earlier, is anticipated to improve the dossier submission as it provides features which will enhance dossier review and help in tagging, hyper-linking and life cycle management of drug etc. Thus, discussion of adoption of eCTD based on the ICH CTD has been initiated in ASEAN. As a result, Thailand is the first country to have adopted eCTD but is yet to assess its benefits. This has also kick started the discussions at the HSA and given the efficiency and highly competent staff at HSA, eCTD might show commendable results.

After PRISM and dossier submission, the application is screened to ensure that the correct application type has been chosen and that there are no deficiencies that would delay the registration process. Such as, if the application type needs to be re-categorised from NDA-2 to NDA-3 or GDA-1 to NDA-2, the applicant will be notified.[59] After the applicant's response is received, it is screened for completeness and henceforth the dossier will be accepted.

The registration process explained here is depicted in the above flowchart (see Figure 3.10) and the timelines for dossier evaluation by the HSA are shown in Table 3.3.

Table 3.3

Approval Timelines of Health Sciences Authority

Screening timeline	*25 working days before the first communication, in the form of an input request or acceptance/non-acceptance notification, is issued*		
Evaluation timeline	Dossier type	NDA	GDA
	Full	270	
	Abridged	180	240
	Verification	60	120
	Verification– CECA		90

Source: *Guidance on Medicinal Product Registration in Singapore*, Health Science Authority, 2011.

57. Unlike what is popular in the literature, as per some of the respondents, ACTD format was developed based on earlier European format and ASEAN had started working on it before the ICH CTD was launched.

58. For example CPPs, approval letters not available online, authorisation letters, GMP certificate, patent declaration, declaration letters, etc.

59. The stop-clock starts whenever HSA requests for clarification or additional information and ends when HSA receives a complete and satisfactory response to the query.

With regard to review of application, HSA has a systemic process with clear communications from time to time and strict adherence to timelines. Other than approval and rejection, decision like approvable and non-approvable is also given in case there are deficiencies in the application which can be corrected by the applicant and submitted again. A study by Wong (2003) analysed data on six new drugs registered in five ASEAN countries, and the results showed approvals were the fastest in Singapore among the five countries, of which Thailand, Indonesia, Philippines and Malaysia were a part.

The above discussion makes a case for Singapore as an attractive destination for MNCs due to reasons such as suitable environment for early drug discovery and manufacturing of biomedical products, efficient and transparent registration system provided by the health regulatory body etc. This can be substantiated by the analysis[60] of new drug approval data in Singapore between 2010-2016 which shows that significantly high number of NDAs have been approved (NDA here includes NDA 1, NDA 2 and NDA 3 together) (See Figure 3.11).

Table 3.4

Category-wise NDA and their Description as per Health Sciences Authority

Type of NDA	*Description*
NDA 1	New chemical or new biological entity (NCE/NBE)
NDA 2	A new combination of registered chemical or biological entities
	Registered chemical or biological entity(ies) in a new dosage form
	Registered chemical or biological entity(ies) for use by a new route of administration
	Registered chemical or biological entity(ies) for new indication(s), dosage recommendation(s) and/or patient population(s)
NDA 3	Subsequent strength(s) of a new drug product that has been registered or has been submitted as an NDA-1 or NDA-2

Source: *Guidance on Medicinal Product Registration in Singapore, Health Science Authority, 2011.*

A noteworthy initiative by HSA has been reporting of category wise approval data since April, 2015 which helps to directly segregate the type of drug approved (NDA 1, NDA 2 or NDA 3). Refer to Table 3.4 for description of category wise NDAs.

60. Data obtained from HSA website. See *http://www.hsa.gov.sg/content/hsa/en/Health_Products_Regulation/Western_Medicines/New_Drug_Approvals.html* (Last accessed on 12 January 2017).

Figure 3.11

Total NDA Approvals

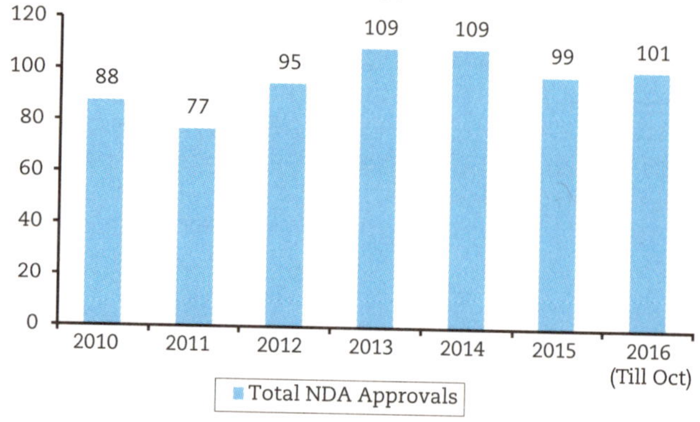

Source: Authors' compilation from list provided at HSA's website.

Figure 3.12

Category-wise NDA Approval (since April 2015)

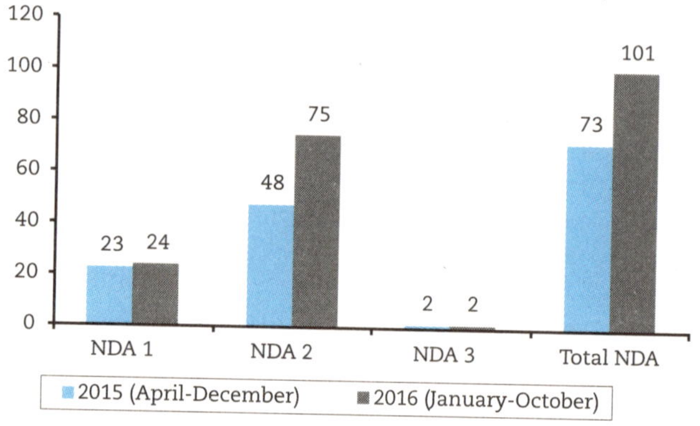

Source: Authors' compilation from list provided at HSA's website.

For analysis as shown in Figure 3.12, we consider the following definitions for NDA 1 and NDA 2. When an additional dosage (NDA 2) or an additional strength (NDA 3) of a drug is approved along with its application for NDA 1, then the said approval is only counted as NDA 1 approval. Also, when an additional strength (NDA 3) and NDA 2 application for a drug are approved together, then it is only counted as NDA 2. The graph shows that NDA 2 product types mainly dominates the approval list and a considerable number of NDA 1 product approvals which amount to 23 and 24 respectively in 2015 (April-December) and 2016 (January-October). But as the data does not cover a significant period of time, it is difficult to analyse the nature of drugs approved. In the long run, this data would be useful in analysing the number of NCEs/NBEs approved and therefore provide insight into the new treatment options brought into the country. Public health impact can be examined through these measures as more number of NDA 1 would mean introduction of new drugs into a class where none existed before that or an advanced treatment has been introduced (NDA 2 approvals only show new dosage/combination/indications introduced of an already registered product). Thus, although it is difficult to derive meaningful conclusions as of now, yet such detailed reporting on drugs approved in the country is a step in the right direction by the HSA.

3.4.2.3 International Cooperation

Being a small country, it is seen as an economic imperative for Singapore to develop international relationships and cooperate with other countries. Nonetheless, its progress cannot be attributed solely to this factor. The drive of the government, political will and stability has made it a centre for trade, research and development and healthcare, which has attracted many companies to this country. In the pharmaceuticals sector, the dearth of a local industry has also added impetus towards its drive to cooperate internationally, adopt global standards and attract MNCs.

Singapore has been one of the most active member states in the ASEAN PPWG groups. It has transposed ASEAN guidelines in its national laws and works effectively to promote cooperation. It is also a part of many other significant initiatives such as ICMRA, PIC/s, APEC and IGDRP—all working on the principle of collaboration and harmonisation. It was also observed that due to sovereignty issues that arise with harmonisation, regulatory convergence is the concept that is of late gaining popularity in this region, and is also being focused on by APEC[61] and IGDRP. In Singapore, HSA along with ASEAN and Centre of Regulatory Excellence (CoRE) at the Duke-National University of Singapore has been focusing on convergence along with harmonisation to improve regulatory practice.[62]

Due to its faster growing pharmaceutical industry, Singapore believes in implementing globally agreed upon scientific guidelines. It has a drive to learn from the expertise of developed regulatory agencies, to be at par with the international best practices and thus add to existing research and science. This has driven it to collaborate with ICH and thus HSA is an observer at the ICH and has adopted many of its guidelines.[63]

In addition to ASEAN harmonisation initiative, Singapore has also cooperated with other countries through various agreements. In regards to registration of drug, Singapore's CECA scheme is a notable step for faster introduction of Indian generics into their markets. Prior to this, Indian drug manufacturers could not export generic drugs to Singapore without undergoing clearances. However, under this new agreement, if the US, EU, Canada, or Australia have approved the Indian drug, then it will not need any more clearances to enter the Singaporean market.[64] This agreement focuses on liberalising the bilateral flow of goods, services and investment. It is a part of the larger initiative to strengthen India—Singapore relations and build connectivity through harmonisation of trade rules and standards (Yong and Bhattacharya 2016).

Besides the above initiatives, HSA is also progressively participating in cooperation initiatives and thus has signed a number of MoUs.[65] An MoU for parallel evaluation has been signed with regulatory authorities of Canada, Switzerland and Australia (Health Canada, Swiss Medic and TGA respectively). The aim was to move from here to joint evaluation in order to reduce duplication of efforts (Lakkis 2010). This consortium, now known as Australia-Canada-Singapore-Switzerland (ACSS) working group, works on generic drug review as a priority area for collaboration for the availability of generic drugs through convergence.[66] Ultimately, the aim is to provide faster access to generic drugs for patients (NEX2US Newsletter 2014, HSA).[67] Among many other MoUs, the ones that include but are not limited to,

61. APEC aims to achieve regional convergence on regulatory approval procedures for medical products by 2020.
62. See *https://www.adb.org/sites/default/files/publication/184392/better-regulation-medicine.pdf* (Last accessed on 13 April 2017).
63. Such as adoption of ICH CTD due to which 53 per cent of dossiers are submitted at HSA in ICH format. See *http://www.ich.org/fileadmin/Public_Web_Site/Meetings/C-GCG_Reports/Nov_2008_Brussels/DRA_Singapore_Presentation_in_Brussels.pdf* (Last accessed on 13 April 2017).
64. *http://www.pacificbridgemedical.com/resource-center/?cat_resource_market=0&_type=news_brief* (Last accessed on 13 April 2017).
65. Its MoU partners include the UK's Medicines and Healthcare Products Regulatory Agency (MHRA), US' Food and Drug Administration, Health Canada's Health Products and Food Branch, Australia's Therapeutic Goods Administration, China's State Food and Drug Administration, Switzerland's Swiss Medic, Sweden's Medical Products Agency etc.
66. The working group aims to share assessment reports, joint reviews and staff exchanges and to eventually establish an effective network among trusted, like-minded regulatory authorities See *https://www.tga.gov.au/australia-canada-singapore-switzerland-acss-consortium* (Last accessed on 13 April 2017).
67. *http://www.hsa.gov.sg/content/dam/HSA/Publications/Nexus/NEX2US_January2014.pdf* (Last accessed on 13 April 2017).

drug registration and approvals are with Malaysia and Korea. These MoUs focus on exchange of regulatory information, work sharing and collaborations in areas of regulatory science.[68, 69]

In conclusion, Singapore, with its capabilities for research on new drugs, a number of research institutions and major pharmaceutical companies combined with HSA's efficient guidelines can serve as a good model if all countries in ASEAN were to harmonise their systems.

3.4.3 Indonesia

3.4.3.1 Brief Background on Medicine Regulation

Indonesia is home to 247 million people, making it the largest country in the ASEAN region in terms of population (40.58%).[70]. However, it is one of the lowest spending nations with respect to healthcare with a per capita total health expenditure of 99 USD in 2014.[71] Although government health expenditure has increased in recent years, total health expenditure has remained below 3 per cent of Gross Domestic Product (GDP). As a consequence of insufficient, inefficient expenditure and shortage of equipment and medicines, the health status of the Indonesian population is poor. To give direction and provide guidance on medicines for the purpose of health development, the National Medicines Policy[72] was drawn up by Indonesia in 1983 and revised in 2006. Its objectives include availability of drugs according to the needs of the population, improve accessibility and affordability and to ensure the efficacy, safety, quality and validity of marketed drugs. The policy also focuses on globalisation, effects of international trade on pharmaceutical products and harmonisation of technical specifications in medicines control and administration, among other important issues. For regulation of drugs, the National Agency for Drug and Food Control (NADFC), an independent body that reports to the President and coordinates with the Ministry of Health, was formed in 2000. It is the national regulator in Indonesia responsible for the provision of safe, effective and high quality medicines to its population by drawing up and implementing policies in the field of supervision of drugs.

Indonesia's pharmaceutical market has historically been dominated by local drugs manufactured by Indonesia-based producers covering 70 per cent of the market with almost 60 foreign pharmaceutical companies control the remaining 30 per cent.[73] There have been growing concerns regarding the high prices of branded generics and the increased risk of entry of counterfeits, coupled with high out-of-pocket expenses and lax enforcement of regulations within the sector. This poses major limitations for the efficient functioning of the sector in spite of Indonesia's tremendous market size and potential. In addition, foreign pharmaceutical companies face several roadblocks in the Indonesian market as a number of laws protect local industry from foreign competition. Decree 1010 has, since 2008, required that all pharmaceuticals registered in the country be locally produced.[74] Hence, foreign drug companies have responded to Decree 1010 by partnering with domestic or other international companies or expanding their own local manufacturing capacity in Indonesia.[75] With regards to the testing of generics, NADFC, in its 2011 decree, issued regulation for equivalence testing of generic products for registration and renewed registration.[76] This helps to guarantee the equivalence of generic products and their original innovators or approved comparators. It also includes the list of products requiring bioequivalence testing (Health Sector Review 2014).[77]

68. For details see *http://www.hsa.gov.sg/content/hsa/en/News_Events/Press_Releases/2012/hsa_signs_memorandum.html* (Last accessed on 15 April 2017).

69. For details See *http://www.hsa.gov.sg/content/hsa/en/News_Events/Press_Releases/2010/hsa_signs_memorandum.html* (Last accessed on 15 April 2017).

70. See *https://aseanup.com/?s=population* (Last accessed on 15 February 2017).

71. World Bank Statistics, 2013. See *http://data.worldbank.org/indicator/SH.XPD.PCAP* (Last accessed on 15 April 2017).

72. See *http://apps.who.int/medicinedocs/documents/s21583en/s21583en.pdf* (Last accessed on 15 April 2017).

73. See *http://www.pacificbridgemedical.com/publication/indonesian-pharmaceuticals-2014-update/* (Last accessed on 15 April 2017).

74. A drug is allowed to be imported only if it falls in one of the following drug categories: for a public health programme, newly invented drug and if a drug cannot be produced locally.

75. See *http://www.pacificbridgemedical.com/regulatory-services/pharmaceutical/product-registration/others/* (Last accessed on 15 April 2017).

76. However, it is not clear how this regulation is being implemented at present, including identification of laboratories needed to undertake such testing and hence, the implications for final cost of the product is unknown. These issues need to be considered to avoid delay in the registration process

77. See *http://aiphss.org/wp-content/uploads/2015/02/Pharmaceutical-Review-and-Medical-Technology.pdf* (Last accessed on 15 April 2017).

Figure 3.13

Drug Registration Process in Indonesia

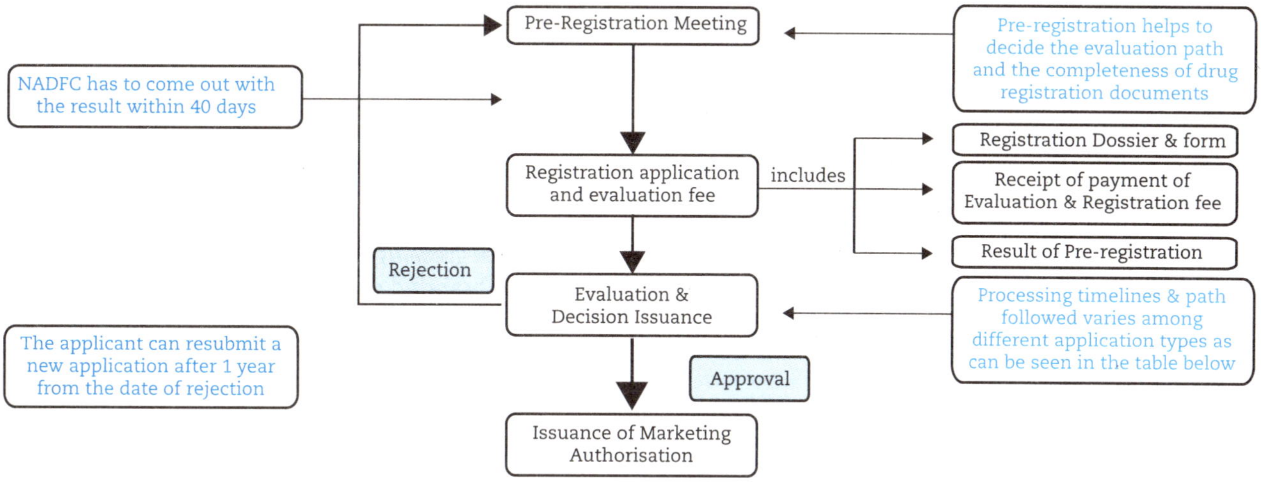

Source: Compiled by authors.

3.4.3.2 Registration Process (Including submission and review processes, approval times, etc)

As recently as in 2011, Indonesia revised regulations for drug registration by introducing the Decree of the Head of the NADFC.[78] Drug approval in Indonesia is a two-staged process: i) pre-registration and ii) submission of registration dossier. The pre-registration is conducted to decide the evaluation path and the NADFC has to come out with its decision within 40 days. Subsequent to the submission of the registration dossier, approval timelines could vary depending upon the category of the drug (see Table 3.5) and it can take as few as 40 working days to as many as 300 working days. Pre-registration meetings help in consultation and in obtaining additional documents needed before the application is processed. Regulators and industry respondents consider this to be an extremely beneficial step in the process of drug registration. This may take a longer time but once the queries are answered, the rest of the process is simplified and efficient.

The drug registration process in Indonesia is depicted in the Figure 3.13 and the timelines for evaluation by the NADFC are stated in Table 3.5.

Table 3.5

Timelines for Drug Registration in Indonesia

		Drug Category	*Time for Approval (working days)*
Path 1	Orphan drugs/drugs for life threatening diseases/ Generic essential drugs for public health program.	Category 1	100
Path 2	New drugs already approved in certain other countries	Category 2	150
Path 3	Others that do not qualify in the above two categories	Category 3	300

Source: Criteria and Procedure of Drug Registration, NADFC.[79]

NADFC allows application submissions for new or copy drugs[80] to be made in ACTD format, which is used throughout ASEAN region with country specific requirements.[81] Due to the benefits associated with

78. See *http://www.flevin.com/id/lgso/translations/JICA%20Mirror/english/4886_HK.03.1.23.10.11.08481_e.html* (Last accessed on 15 April 2017).

79. See more at *http://apps.who.int/medicinedocs/documents/s18009en/s18009en.pdf* (Last accessed on 15 April 2017).

80. New drug or new finished drug is a drug, which contains a new active ingredient or composition or dosage from/route of administration or indication or posology that has not been approved in Indonesia. Copy drug or finished 'me too' drug is a drug which contain the same active ingredients as a registered drug. Definition as per Decree of the head of NADFC Republic of Indonesia.

81. Country-specific requirements refer to package size, registration number, name and industry address, expiry date, source of available raw materials, methods and test result of stability/durability etc.

a common format of the dossier, authorities in Indonesia have adopted the ACTD format in the right spirit along with other ASEAN countries. During our field interactions, regulators said that it facilitates filing of dossier and enhances review capabilities. It has also reduced the resources needed to change the dossiers every time a company has to apply to ASEAN countries. In order to analyse the drug approvals in the country, we examined the data from a recent list of total drugs (new and copy drugs) provided by NADFC.[82] On assessing the figures from 2010-2016 (see column 2 in Table 3.6), it was observed that a significantly large number of drugs are approved each year, with the number being as high as 2286 in 2015. But the list does not uncover the NDA approvals in the country as there is no demarcation between a copy drug[83] and a new drug. However on exploring an old dataset[84] provided by NADFC, which displays only the number of new drugs approved, we find that this figure is very minor—as low as 10 in the year 2013 (column 3 in the table) as compared with the total drugs approved, which is 2190 in the same year (column 2 in the table).

Table 3.6

Drugs Approved in Indonesia (2010-2016)[85]

Year	*Total Drugs Approved (New Drugs and Copy Drugs)*	*New Drugs Approved*
2016	1993	
2015	2286	-
2014	1499	-
2013	2190	10
2012	1982	27
2011	1287	22
2010	1231	43

Source: Authors' compilation from list provided at NADFC's website.

Thus, the probabilistic view—that can be comprehended from the above data—is that the difference between the 2 columns shows the number of copy drugs approved in the country. The total drugs data also counts different dosages of a drug that, although approved together, feature as separate entries in the list which further increases its number. Consequently, this analysis supports the argument that Indonesia is mainly a producer of copy drugs and the approvals of new drugs are less in the country.

3.4.3.3 Issues and Concerns

ACTD has been successful in harmonising the submission format but there is no evidence that suggests that its use has brought about reductions in review times. Additionally, the existence of country specific requirements among ASEAN member states act as hurdles in registration. A study by Wong (2003) analysed data on six NCEs in five ASEAN Countries (Singapore, Malaysia, Thailand, Indonesia and Philippines) and found that it took a longer time than stated for approvals in Indonesia. Thus the issue of delays in approvals is a cause of concern in Indonesia as expressed during field interaction as well. The failure to follow the timelines is mainly linked to the lack of technical expertise within the health authority. There is an increase in the number of applications which is not supplemented by an enhanced availability of resources and capacity, leading to uncertainty in approvals.

A more recent analysis by Liberti et al. (2012) shows that while the submission gap in Indonesia is lower than that in India, the time taken for granting approval is greater. Besides, in Indonesia, as in many other countries, approvals are based upon prior approvals by advanced countries. This is done through their reliance on free sales certificate or CPP, which has to be submitted with the dossier. Wong (2003) states that the requirement of CPP from the country of origin (COO) is a key barrier to the registration of drugs in these countries as it delays the registration to the point until the drug is launched in the reference countries and the certificate is made available. However, during field interactions, we learnt that CPP is considered to fast track the registration process in countries like Indonesia as the regulatory bodies do not have the capacity and scientific knowhow to conduct a full evaluation of the dossier. In such instances, it can give the regulator an assurance of the drug and they can fast track the process. Without the CPP, there can be significant delays in drug approvals in Indonesia.

In order to further enhance the review process in Indonesia, regional ties and joint assessments are suggested as the way forward. This will not only help

82. The list can be accessed at *http://ceknie.pom.go.id/index.php/home/produk/8a8e73cda792d863de1426b1f118b9d2/01* (Last accessed on 30 December 2016).

83. Copy Drug here includes: Copy drug with trade names and Copy Drug with generic names.

84. Data not updated after year 2013.

85. New drugs approval data can be accessed at *http://www.pom.go.id/index.php/io/menu/03/obat/2013/1*. Total drugs approved can be accessed at *http://ceknie.pom.go.id/index.php/home/produk/8a8e73cda792d863de1426b1f118b9d2/01* (Last accessed on 30 December 2016).

in faster approvals but also enhance the regulatory capacity of the government by learning from experts at mature jurisdictions. Further, lack of transparency and communication between the regulator and industry is highlighted as a major concern and a need for a stronger interface between them is required. Also, data analysis in Indonesia highlighted that it will be useful if new drug approvals and its further categories are listed separately by NADFC as currently new and copy drugs data is provided together without demarcation. This information will help in conducting useful analysis about new or advanced treatment being brought in Indonesia and the therapeutic areas covered. Thus, such information will help in evaluating the public health impact in the country which is currently difficult to achieve.

3.4.3.4 International Cooperation

In its attempts at harmonising with ASEAN standards, Indonesia had adopted the ACTD format and ACTR completely by 2007.[86] This has made it easy for the health authority to review the dossier as only one format is being followed. In the case of MRA on GMP, there has not been much progress on the ground although it has been implemented in theory. It was observed during field interactions that due to lack of expertise, inspections done by Indonesia may not be trusted by other countries.[87]

Even though efforts towards harmonisation are perceived positively in this country, progress has been slow. Indonesia presents a contrasting picture to Singapore in the degree of success, even though both are a part of ASEAN harmonisation. A significant country and population size as compared to Singapore, coupled with the domination of the local pharmaceutical industry focused on production of generics, is one of the main reasons for this. The local industry shows scepticism towards harmonisation initiatives as it would attract more foreign companies and increase the level of standards and guidelines that would have to be followed. However as stated during the field interviews, more recently, harmonisation is being regarded as a means to improve the quality of medicines which lies in the interest of public health. It would also pave the path for export of drugs. With ease in access to Indonesia markets, there will be an increase in imports, which will also bring in new and quality drugs along with research and innovation which, at present, is absent in the country.

3.5 South Africa

3.5.1 *Brief Background of Medicine Regulations*

Medicines and Related Substances Act (Act 101 of 1965) regulates and controls medicines, scheduled substances and medical devices, as well as licences for manufacturing, storage and distribution facilities within South Africa. Under the provisions of the Act, the Medical Control Council (MCC) was formed in 1966 as the primary regulatory body for medicines. The MCC oversees the ethical evaluation and registration of medicines; including NCEs, generic products, product line extensions, and biological medicines; undertakes periodic assessments and monitoring, undertakes inspections and audits to check compliance with regulations and regulates CTs.[88]

In 2007, the Pharmaceutical Manufacturing Plan for Africa was conceived by the African Union Commission to strengthen the ability of African member states to produce high quality and affordable medicines that contribute towards improved health outcomes and provide direct and indirect economic benefits. Thereafter, in 2008, the report of Ministerial Task Team observed that, like many developing countries, MCC had capacity shortages that resulted in huge backlog of drug approvals. The problem was further compounded by low remuneration of part-time evaluators and the consequent poor retention of skilled regulatory staff (Matsebula et al. 2005). Recently, to widen the regulatory landscape, the Medicines and Related Substances Amendment Act of 2015 has been passed allowing the South African Health Products Regulatory Authority (SAHPRA) to replace the MCC.

3.5.2 *Registration Process*

Before placing a medicine in the South African market, an application[89] for registration of medicines

86. ACTD came into force in 2003 but countries were given time to adopt it completely.

87. Even though PIC/S has multiple countries participating in it, but it is challenging for developing countries as they feel that their reviews may not be considered at par with those of the developed ones. Developed countries would be sceptical of the inspections and approvals given by developing countries and thus an equal footing relation can't be established.

88. Please see: *http://www.kznhealth.gov.za/research/mccinfo.pdf* (Last accessed on 13 April 2017).

89. The applicant is required to be registered and operating in South Africa, and must be registered with South African Pharmacy Council.

Figure 3.14

Drug Registration Process in South Africa

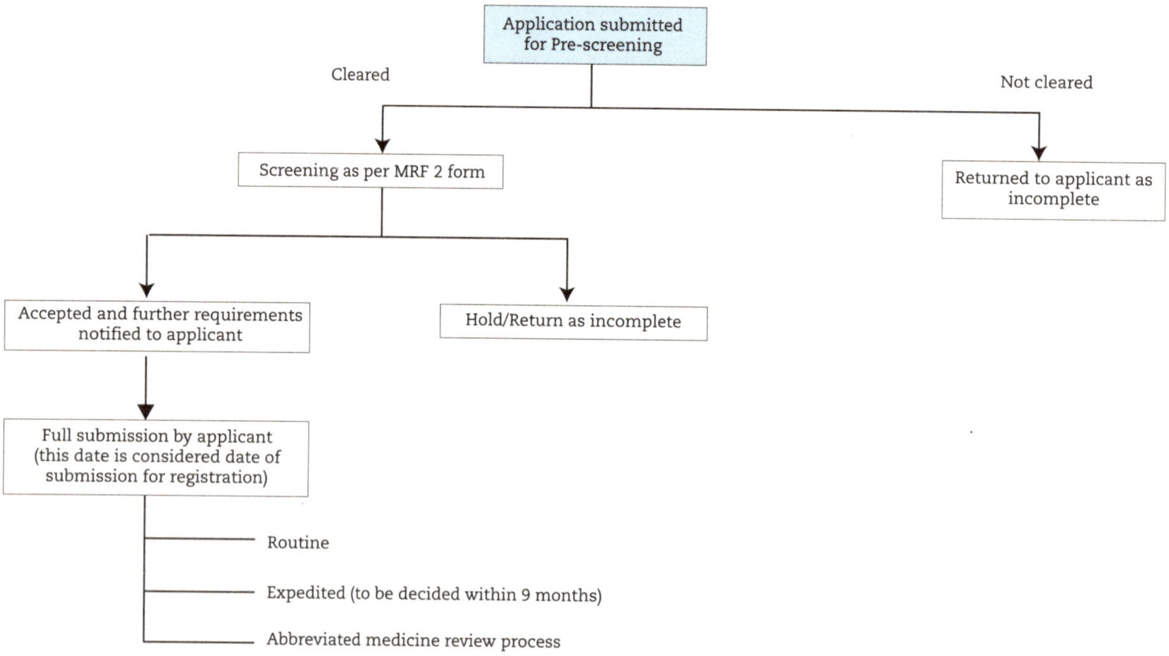

Source: Compiled by authors.

(refer to Figure 3.14) is reviewed by the MCC, which assesses the drug on the basis of quality, safety and efficacy. The first step is to hold a pre-registration consultation meeting between the applicant and the regulator, to address issues related to the development of the drug. When the applicant is ready to register the drug, he must first submit a set of documents for the pre-screening process which is evaluated as per a checklist of documents. Upon being cleared, the application is then screened in order to confirm that all data has been included and doesn't involve evaluation of either the data or any motivation for omission of data. Subsequent to its acceptance at this stage, the MCC notifies the applicant to make a full submission along with the application fee. The date of the final submission is considered as the date of registration and the review process begins with the MCC appointing expert committees that are asked to consider parts of the applications such as pre-clinical and clinical data, pharmaceutical and analytical data and clinical trials. So while one committee looks into the clinical data, another will recommend the 'scheduling status' of the medicine i.e. whether it is to be made available as a prescription only drug or not.[90] Since the dossiers for innovator products are generally first submitted to advanced jurisdictions, an abbreviated medicine review process[91] is available for which the MCC aligns itself with the following authorities: the United States Food and Drug Administration (USFDA), the United Kingdom's Medicines and Healthcare Products Regulatory (MHRA), Sweden's Medical Products Agency (MPA), Australia's Therapeutic Goods Administration (TGA), Canada's Health Canada, EU's European Medicines Agency (EMEA) and Japan's Ministry of Health, Labour and Welfare (MHLW). For medicines on the Essential Drug List (EDL) or those NCEs considered essential for national health but do not appear on the EDL, there's an expedited review process in which the MCC has to come out with a decision within 9 months. All other drugs go through the routine review, but this has no statutory timeline.

Regarding registration of generics, there are two distinct provisions in South Africa. First, BE data can be submitted to demonstrate safety and efficacy; the comparator product need not necessarily be of

90. Health and Democracy, Section 27, 2007 available at *http://section27.org.za/wp-content/uploads/2010/04/Chapter13.pdf* (Last accessed on 13 April 2017).

91. This is applicable for cases where the product has been approved by these authorities in the past three years and the evaluation report is available (Parsons et al. 2015).

domestic origin (Kanfer et al. 2016).[92] Second, the registration of generics is allowed before patent expiration. Besides, to curb abuse of patent rights and increase access to cheaper and good quality medicines, South Africa has a provision for parallel imports and compulsory licensing (Matsebula et al. 2005, Parsons et al. 2015).

3.5.3 Issues and Concerns

A growing concern in South Africa is one with respect to essential medicines.[93] Since all medicines in the essential medicines list (which includes mostly generics) as well as all NCEs are eligible for a fast track review, it has a tendency to clog the system and slacken the process of review. As a result, it takes considerably longer than the nine month registration decision timeline that the fast track system provides. Leng et al. (2016) and Leng et al. (2015) point out that the backlog includes routine applications (other than fast track) received up to December 2011 (since the MCC's strategy for allocation of applications has been to look at those received between January and March 2012) and these would only be evaluated once the MCC has the requisite additional capacity to begin reviewing them. According to the minutes of the latest Industry Task Group meeting held in March 2016[94], we now know that the MCC is currently evaluating routine applications that were submitted between June-August 2012 and issuing screening outcome letters for applications that were submitted up to August/ September 2014. This suggests that the backlog issue has only been amplified by other shortcomings such as the insufficiency of skilled manpower and poor infrastructure at the MCC (as indicated by Leng et al. 2016).

92. However, it is argued that BE based on a foreign reference product may not be interchangeable and generic substitution has shown to be an acceptable equivalent only in case the domestic innovator product is used as the reference (or comparator) (ibid).

93. As per the National Drug Policy for South Africa—essential drugs are drugs that are required to treat the majority of conditions that are prevalent in a country in a cost-effective and efficient manner. The concept does not imply that no other drugs are useful, but that these drugs are the most needed for the health care of the majority of the population. They should therefore be available at all times, in adequate amounts and in the proper dosage forms. For further details, see *http://apps.who.int/medicinedocs/documents/s17744en/s17744en.pdf* (Last accessed on 13 April 2017).

94. Industry Task Group Meeting held on 8 March 2016 available at *http://www.mccza.com/documents/9791ec502016_03_08_Final_ITG_meeting_minutes.pdf* (Last accessed on 9 September 2016).

To gauge the volume of applications that come to the MCC, we consider the trends based on data provided by Leng et al. (2015). As evident from Figure 3.15, albeit a dip in 2010, the number of applications being made to the MCC is increasing each year and a lion's share of these are generic medicine applications.

Figure 3.15

Trends in Registration of Medicines in South Africa

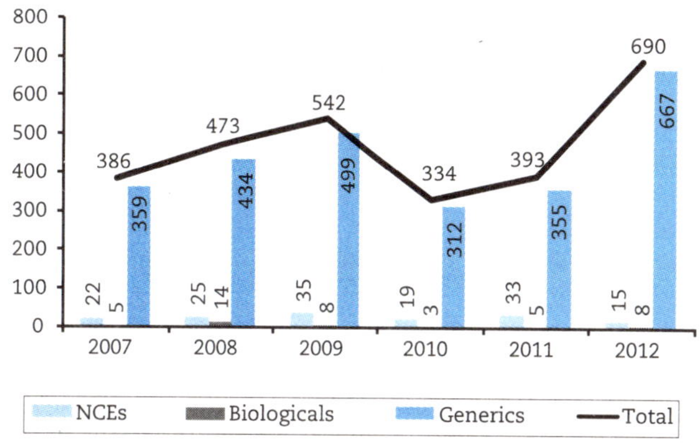

Source: Adapted from data provided by Leng et al. (2015).

Additionally, Leng et al. (2015) shows that there is a large number of duplicate GDAs i.e. applications made by the same manufacturer under different brand names. During our field interactions, we were told that this has become a common practice in South Africa for two reasons, one, to mitigate the process of delayed registrations and second, because of the policy of a single exit price i.e. same price for all sellers regardless of volume. By submitting multiple dossiers for multiple brand names containing the same chemical compound, the applicant can treat the licence as an asset that can be sold off later. Further, due to the policy of a single exit price, if any manufacturers wanted to segment the market, he/she would have to sell the same drug under different brand names to buyers with different purchase volumes.

To explore more recent data since 2012, we examined the list of new drugs provided by the MCC on their website. We find that in 2013, 2014 and 2015, the total number of drug registrations were—648,467, 689, respectively. However those lists do not provide useful information that could throw some light as to whether the registered drugs are NCEs, biologicals or generics. This severely limits our ability to do a meaningful analysis of the data. We, however, did note a continued trend of duplicate entries of generic drugs.

3.5.4 International Cooperation

While the South African industry has been using the CTD format for export purposes for a long time now, it was made compulsory for submission of an application to the MCC, only in 2011. South Africa's MCC brought in CTD in order to bring about greater harmonisation by providing for a common format of submission of information in the ICH regions and South Africa.[95] Recognising that this format does not ensure harmonisation of content, the advantages it seeks come from facilitation of simultaneous submissions in all regions, exchange of regulatory information and more efficient assessment and navigation through the use of hyperlinks and bookmarks. In an attempt to further harmonise the submission format, the MCC eCTD submission went live in April 2016 for NCEs and it is envisaged this facility will be available for generics by January 2017. Meanwhile, the agency is still grappling with establishing the eCTD framework and the technical specifications of the applications, in particular.

To assist African nations to strengthen regulatory capacity and to harmonise medicine registration, a conference organised by New Partnership for Africa's Development (NEPAD) and the Pan African Parliament (PAP) in 2009 marked the genesis of the AMRH initiative. It aims to improve public health by increasing rapid access to safe and effective medicines of good quality for the treatment of priority diseases; it also aims to reduce the time taken to register essential medicines.[96] The AMRH initiative works with various Regional Economic Communities (RECs)[97] to fulfil the vision of the pharmaceutical manufacturing plan for Africa. So far the AMRH has made proposals to and begun work with the southern and eastern RECs and will shortly be beginning work on the western RECs as well.

South Africa is also a part of an REC i.e. the Southern African Development Community (SADC) which comprises about 15 member states[98] in the southern African region. However, SADC has not done particularly well on the medicines regulatory harmonisation front so far as compared with its eastern counterpart, the East African Community (EAC). This is mainly because the member states within SADC are at quite different levels of development which is not the case with the EAC, which consists of five countries that are more or less similar. Over the years, the MCC's involvement in the SADC region has also reduced—which regulatory experts believe, is due to the mismatch in regulatory capacities given that the MCC is the most powerful regulator in the region. While South Africa could not harmonise downwards, it doesn't want to take a leadership role in the region since all participating authorities are considered as equals in the group.

Within the SADC region, one particular initiative has gained much popularity—ZAZIBONA—a collaboration of Zambia, Zimbabwe, Namibia and Botswana. According to the AMRH NEPAD Newsletter,[99] South Africa has recently joined the ZAZIBONA initiative, although there seems no official announcement from the MCC. The success of the ZAZIBONA model stems from the way it is structured as a collaborative network among similarly resourced regulators. None of these four countries have particularly strong regulatory authorities and by coming together to do joint assessments, they are pooling in their limited resources and in the process, strengthening their systems as well. These four countries meet about four times a year to evaluate common applications and conduct their reviews under the supervision of an expert from the WHO. While this centralised system does not have a provision for a single submission for all countries, it does allow submission of single dossier based on the SADC CTD in each of the countries. In addition, the end result of the ZAZIBONA programme is not to register the product but instead, only to give a recommendation and it is upto the individual member states to decide whether or not they want to register the product in their respective countries. Although, this is a rare event,

95. 'Get Ready for eCTD in South Africa: Current status at MCC' Estelle Tautee, February 2013 available at *http://www.mccza.com/documents/a8cf28deeCTD_current_status_14-15_Feb2013E_Taute.pdf* (Last accessed on 9 September 2016).

96. See *http://apps.who.int/medicinedocs/documents/s20130en/s20130en.pdf* (Last accessed on 15 April 2017).

97. The RECs in Africa are not only building blocks for economic integration in Africa but also, in collaboration with the African Union, play an instrumental role in maintaining peace and stability within their respective regions. There are 8 RECs recognised by the African Union viz. the Arab Maghreb Union (UMA), Economic Community of West African States (ECOWAS), East African Community (EAC), Inter-governmental Authority on Development (IGAD), Southern African Development Community (SADC), Common Market for Eastern and Southern Africa (COMESA), Economic Community of Central African States (ECCAS) and the Community of Sahel-Saharan States (CENSAD).

98. SADC includes the following member states; Angola, Botswana, Democratic Republic of Congo, Lesotho, Madagascar, Malawi, Mauritius, Mozambique, Namibia, Seychelles, South Africa, Swaziland, United Republic of Tanzania, Zambia, Zimbabwe.

99. The AMRH Newsletter June 2016 is available at *http://www.nepad.org/resource/african-medicines-regulatory-harmonisation-newsletter-june-2016* (Last accessed on 15 April 2017).

but in case a country chooses not to register the product, it is expected to provide its due reasons. The programme has been doing quite well and so far 105 products have been reviewed. Of these, 28 products have been registered.

Other initiatives towards international cooperation of registration of medicines include MCC's membership at a number of international forums such as ICMRA, PIC/S, and IGDRP. Recently MCC has joined the ranks of an observer at the ICH. Besides, MCC has an MOU with Swissmedic which has been instrumental in setting up the CTD framework in South Africa.

While these initiatives are taking place across the African region, it is important to take cognizance of the fact that there is a strong need for internal restructuring in the absence of which it will not be possible for countries to really be able to address the larger public health goal. There is some recognition of this fact within South Africa, since the MCC has not shown much involvement in SADC or AMRH in general, given that it is at a critical juncture where it needs to address its domestic issues on an urgent basis. In this regard, the transformation of the MCC to SAPHRA is envisaged to be the game changer for the South African drug regulatory landscape.

4

Cross-Country Implications for Stakeholders

At first, while it should be noted that there is no-one-size-fits-all policy that can be chosen as a successful formula for streamlining regulatory pathways (countries choose strategies that best suit their local requirements—as has been elucidated in the previous section), due cognizance needs to be taken of the interdependencies between these pathways, as well.

Given these pathways, it may be noted that the impact of regulatory diversity differs across economic sectors, affecting highly export oriented sectors more than import competing ones.[1] Further, regulatory convergence across countries critically requires that firms in different political jurisdictions have interests in a common regulatory standard and that consumers are unopposed to these standards as well.[2] The absence of these crucial requirements, may lead to greater divergences in policies across countries, thereby doing away with any possibility of regulatory convergence.[3]

This section attempts to bring forth the different implications for each stakeholder which could vary across regulatory settings as mentioned in the preceding paragraph. This is done through a detailed analysis of the implications for three set of stakeholders i.e. the patients—which is the public health concern, the industry and regulators, to draw upon lessons from current best practices in select countries.

4.1 Public Health

Processes such as convergence assume importance in the context of addressing the public health goals of a country through multiple channels including increased access to medicines for essential ailments, ensuring production of good quality medicines, reduction of unnecessary testing in animals and humans, and building trust in national health systems (Lezotre 2014). Let's consider each of these individually.

Intuitively speaking, increased access that would follow from a framework of harmonised guidelines would likely facilitate seamless flow of medicines across the region, since firms would have to expend fewer resources (including time resource) in meeting the requirements as they apply for marketing authorisation in different markets. Although, it should be noted that this proposed benefit has not yet been measured in any of the regions that have adopted harmonised guidelines. Moreover, from our field interactions with experts in the EU, the US, Singapore, we learnt that while there has been an increase in innovation in these regions, it may not be possible to attribute measurable gains to such harmonisation alone, as the effect of other regulatory factors like changes in legislations, increased clarity on procedures, etc. could not be isolated. Nevertheless given that harmonised guidelines provide a framework to operate, they do facilitate increased access to global markets.

Indonesia, on the other hand, is yet to realise any measure of success from harmonisation in this sector. Nonetheless, the expected benefits due to harmonisation are touted to be significant. Given that the mainstay has been the generic local industry, cooperating in the global arena will create a regulatory and business environment that has greater potential to attract medical innovation into the country. In addition, the issue with respect to delay in approvals is expected to be resolved through joint assessments and collaborations with competent regulators, further enabling early launch of medicines in the country. These will be beneficial, especially towards addressing unmet medical needs.

Implications emanating specifically from the use of CTD, as per most respondents, were not very clear cut. The industry experts in Singapore, however, did mention that ease of filing in a country impacts their decisions to submit their applications. Therefore, a company would first prepare the dossier in ICH CTD format as a number of countries would be covered in this first round. Subsequently, it would move on to ASEAN region using the common ACTD format and then focus on other countries that use their local formats. Thus, some of respondents were of the view that, a drug is brought early in Singapore as it accepts both the formats (ICH CTD and ACTD), in contrast to other ASEAN countries.

Second, streamlining of regulatory procedures, say through harmonising them in a region, paves the way for legitimate competition that brings in registered medicines that are not fake or substandard. Some of our respondents brought forth instances that in some African countries, a number of products are known

1. Hart (2007).
2. The EU, ASEAN and AMRH initiatives can be seen as illustration of regional cooperation, wherein countries with cultural and structural commonalities as well as relatively similar economic interests, pool their limited resources together to leverage the benefits of harmonisation.
3. An example is the biotechnology sector, where in spite of globalisation, significant divergences in the approach of the US and the EU has impeded the process of regulatory convergence across developed and developing countries. For details, see Falkner and Gupta (2009).

to bypass the regulatory system and are available in the market without a regulatory approval. This sort of a system also propagates the existence of dual standards i.e. high standards for the export market (intra-African trade) while low standards for the domestic market. In such a scenario, two distinct quality products will prevail in the market and may give rise to the phenomenon of lemonisation as elucidated in George Akerlof's 'market for lemons'. Given that the seller has more information about the product quality than the buyer does, maintaining a low standard is likely to ensure that only lemons are supplied. Here corrective measures or 'anti-lemon devices' may be used to credibly assure quality (Katz 2007). Therefore, if the regulatory environment is more streamlined, such that it attracts legitimate business, then it can be ensured that the drugs that reach the masses are safe and effective.

Third, with acceptance of CT data across regions, there might be reduced testing on animals and humans. However, this is not the scenario in present day context as most countries have requirements for local clinical data that is representative of their own population.

Finally, the judgements regarding safety, quality and efficacy in medicines are not as apparent as they are in most other products. Often, substantially different country requirements and regulatory structures lead to differences in approaches to evaluate the same medicines and at times lead to very different regulatory outcomes as well. This in turn has bearing upon the confidence in health systems, as patients find it extremely disturbing when they see different regulators reaching different conclusions about the same product. Some experts interviewed during our field research were of the opinion that harmonised guidelines and increased interaction among regulators could reduce such discrepancy and in turn increase trust in health systems.

4.2 Regulator

Pharmaceutical regulation in countries has significantly evolved and matured over the years. The role of different ethnicities, socio-cultural dynamics, political environment, and a history of adverse events (like Thalidomide catastrophe) has been instrumental in shaping the domestic standards and regulations. Given that the pharmaceutical sector has increasingly globalised, ranging from increasing multi-regional CTs to registration and launch of safe and quality medicines, regulation has become a costly task for the medicine regulatory authorities.

In this regard, international cooperation initiatives have worked as an important tool in utilisation of limited resources to achieve regulatory objectives. As highlighted in the previous section, multiple pathways towards achieving greater regulatory convergence and cooperation are considered by the regulatory agencies, including, harmonising technical requirements, mutual recognition agreements, information sharing through confidentiality agreements, work sharing through collaborative efforts, etc. Also, with specific reference to medicine registration, while initiatives like ICH and ASEAN PPWG have made efforts to facilitate seamless submissions (in form of CTD), the review processes continue to differ from country to country. This essentially arises from the varying approaches that regulatory bodies adopt to assess each of the parameters—safety, quality and efficacy—of the product.

In terms of participation in international cooperation initiatives, the agenda and the experience of mature regulatory jurisdictions like the US and the EU, is different from that of regulators of developing countries. Stringent regulators like USFDA and EMA have proactively participated and promoted international cooperation through the membership of harmonisation initiatives (such as ICH), entering into confidentiality commitments, MoUs and other cooperative arrangements like reliance on GMP, etc. In the US, since the implementation of the FDA Modernization Act in 1997, the FDA has taken on a mission to "participate through appropriate processes with representatives of other countries to reduce the burden of regulation, harmonise regulatory requirements, and achieve appropriate reciprocal arrangements." Such partnerships have enabled the FDA to develop an information network through which regulators worldwide can also share knowledge about criminal enterprises, as well as leverage the knowledge and resources of trusted counterpart agencies (Lezotre 2014: 166). A similar approach has been adopted even in the EU, and the EMA is proactively involved in bilateral (confidentiality agreements, MRAs in GMP, EU falsified medicines directive, etc.) and multilateral arrangements (in collaboration with WHO, Council for Europe, ICMRA, IPRF, etc.) in addition to the internal EU wide harmonisation process. During our field interactions, it was widely acknowledged that while the process of harmonisation to begin with was trade driven, it has translated into considerable benefits to the regulators in various areas including registration of medicines. The medicine registration procedures facilitate a considerable amount of work sharing between the competent authorities of the member states in Europe. As the medicine dossier evaluation process at EMA requires input from the rapporteur and co-rapporteur appointed by CHMP, this provides a forum for discussions and learning between the different regulatory bodies within the Europe. The confidentiality agreements and harmonised guidelines have facilitated discussions of common substantive issues between the regulators including the parameters to be applied while carrying out assessments, which further enhances the capacity of the regulatory system.

From our field interactions, we learnt that while FDA's work sharing agreements with other regulatory counterparts have begun with inspections,[4] there is hope that in due course this may continue for co-registration opportunities as well. But given the cautiousness with which the USFDA has approached the issue of harmonisation specifically related to approving drugs for marketing in the US, it has been a challenge for them to find a common ground with quite a few developing country regulators. The FDA has seen merit in, and therefore continued to invest in, capacity building initiatives of developing country counterparts, with an expectation that improving other regulators will strengthen FDA's ability to protect the supply of medicine in the US. Towards this end, EMA's approach has been quite proactive and in addition to capacity building initiatives, EMA has made strides in efforts to facilitate registration of medicines outside the EU through Article 58 procedure, and real time sharing of assessment reports of generic products, with non-EU regulators in IGDRP.

International cooperation activities have been a great source of learning for maturing medicine regulatory authorities as well through capacity building and training activities by stringent authorities and WHO, by incorporation of best practices, including those related to good manufacturing, clinical and review practices. The experiences among the developing countries have been largely linked with their domestic priorities and resource constraints. In Africa, harmonisation has been a welcome step for most regulators in the region. However, the South African regulator—MCC, has shown relatively less involvement in the SADC region in the recent past owing to the fact that there is a mismatch between the regulatory capacities in the region coupled with language disparities. Additionally, at present, enabling smooth operationalisation of common guidelines seems challenging due to varying level of expertise of regulators (vis-a-vis MCC) across the region. Nevertheless, the MCC has shown interest in participating at global forums. As mentioned earlier, the MCC is also adopting some of the ICH guidelines, such as the eCTD. Though the MCC did incur some costs of the technical specifications and computers, and an annual maintenance fee that has to be paid, but none of this seems to have imposed a burden on the MCC's budget. It is also providing training to its evaluators as well as to the industry in order to reduce instances of compliance errors. This seems to suggest that while South Africa has been open to adopting international guidelines and frameworks that are likely to enhance regulatory efficiency, but at the same time it has taken cognizance of the limitations that eCTD presents by providing a one way transmission between MCC and the industry (since there is paper based transmission from the MCC to the industry).

In terms of regional harmonisation, ASEAN harmonisation initiative is considered to be a trade driven initiative with PPWG focusing on eliminating technical barriers to trade while ensuring quality, safety and efficacy of products. Though such a regional initiative is expected to benefit the resource constrained authorities, the impact has not been strong and uniform throughout ASEAN due to a number of localised factors. It has been observed that while Singapore is reaping the benefits of a number of cooperation initiatives, the Indonesian regulatory authority is still struggling to even apply ASEAN guidelines completely in the country due to capacity constraints. Singapore is also an observer at the ICH and through its regular participation at the ICH meetings, HSA has sought numerous learning opportunities through such expert interactions. Streamlined regulatory procedures at the HSA is one of the reasons that makes Singapore a favourable destination for MNCs. With research and innovation brought into the country by companies, it has made strides in ensuring timely availability of quality medicines for the public which is the end goal of the regulator. Further, bilateral agreements and MoUs with different regulatory authorities have facilitated joint evaluation, sharing of assessment reports, joint inspections (through MRA on GMP), joint trainings etc. which reduces the duplication of regulatory work, thus time and financial resources. The acceptance

4. Exchange of inspection reports have resulted in saving of considerable resources for the regulator, especially in the context of foreign inspections. Given the costs incurred in carrying out foreign inspections are often enormous, the US FDA significantly benefits from various forms of collaboration, for example—the setting up of local or regional offices of the US FDA.

of ACTD has brought consistency in evaluation and thus facilitated the review process in both Singapore and Indonesia. Further, it is expected that a common application format will enable regulators to collaborate while reviewing and exchanging information.

Going forward, based on the European model, there are discussions on having a Pan-ASEAN registration procedure in the ASEAN region to assist the less advanced countries. To assess future implications for Indonesia, such a registration procedure or joint assessments as discussed through SIAHR, will enable NADFC to learn from the capabilities of the reviewers in mature jurisdictions like Singapore. This will also help address other concerns in Indonesia as well, such as, shortage of in-house expertise and lags in drug approvals. Also, cooperation is projected to bring in newer therapies which are currently unavailable to the local population.

Further, on the lines of the ZAZIBONA initiative, there are discussions around setting up the African Medicine Agency (by 2018), with the aim of pooling technical support and capacities of various countries in the African region, thereby replicating the EMA model. However, based on our field interactions, integrating 54 countries would involve challenges, including lack of common legislation as that of Europe, and large disparities—economic and cultural—between the member countries.

To sum up, while there are many benefits of various ongoing and proposed international cooperation initiatives to the regulators, they are not to substitute the need for strong national regulatory bodies. These initiatives can be explored as opportunities in the direction of strengthening the national regulatory capacities. This is of particular relevance as national sovereignty in the form of regional and country specific requirements continues to be a matter of some concern (Lezotre 2014: 178). Thus, international cooperation and strengthening of regulatory capacities can be seen as mutually reinforcing and complementary rather than mere substitutes for one another.

4.3 Industry

As the pharmaceutical industry is becoming increasingly globalised in nature, possibilities for international cooperation on various aspects of medicine regulation translate into measurable gains for the industry as well. For one, it presents a route to reduce technical barriers to trade, but beyond that it also seeks to lower drug development and launch times due to fewer requirements for duplication of studies. Hence, industry has been a pioneer in the foundation of such cooperation initiatives. In this regard, forums like the ICH and ASEAN are following the pathways of harmonisation and regulatory convergence to reduce the duplication of work, enhance focus on safety, quality and efficacy and protect public health through its impact on the regulator and industry both.

There is considerable influence of international cooperation initiatives on pharmaceutical trade and industry. Hence the ensuing impacts needs to be assessed carefully for the sake of patients and their access to medicines. For example, fulfilling separate requirements in different countries is a challenge for the industry which not only adds to its cost and efforts but also leads to delay in the launch of drugs (Lezotre 2014). As noted previously in this report, the development of the CTD by the ICH (2000) was intended to save time and other resources that companies invest in preparing dossiers for different countries and was expected to result in increased efficiencies.[5] This point was substantiated during our field research as well. CTD has been adopted by countries beyond ICH member nations as well, among which South Africa is an interesting case. In addition to the CTD, its electronic version i.e. the eCTD is also gradually making its way into the country's regulatory system. While this could impose considerable costs on the smaller generic players in South Africa, our industry respondents mentioned that there hasn't been much opposition from the smaller companies in this country. For a number of regulatory services, the smaller players in South Africa already rely on outsourcing and so, the adoption of eCTD will follow the same course and is unlikely to impose significant costs upon them. Likewise, ASEAN's ACTD format has benefitted the industry considerably in this region by reducing the need to duplicate efforts as one dossier can be used across ASEAN countries; however, the country specific requirements have limited actual impact.

Harmonisation initiatives have also enabled an interaction between health authorities and the industry which is channelled through industry

5. Although in the reports by ICH, *The Value and Benefits of ICH to Industry & Drug Regulatory Authorities*, it was anticipated that CTD would revolutionise the submission procedures and simplify the task for the industry, yet from the field interactions we learnt that the benefit has been limited to not having to create separate dossiers. Also, huge country specific requirements still exist in the format.

associations. In ASEAN, APC and APRIA participate in the discussions at ASEAN meetings and are able to put across their concerns at the regional level. APRIA envisages that joint evaluation or MRA on registration, if achieved, will help in faster introduction of drugs in the region. This will help the industry by easing the process of drug launch. Similarly, ICH has created constructive dialogue between regulatory authorities and the industry in identifying the real and perceived differences in the technical requirements for product registration. This is expected to ensure a more timely introduction of new medicinal products for patients in the participating regions (WHO report 2001). The founding members of the ICH include not only the regulators of the three regions, the US, the EU and Japan, but also their respective industry bodies making sure that industry associations work alongside the regulator in all the regions. Also, the ICH has recently included International Generic and Biosimilar Medicines Association (IGBA) (along with other organisations and regulatory agencies) as an industry member to represent generic industry in its harmonisation initiative. This has resulted from an expansion of the focus of the ICH beyond the innovative medicines to include generic medicines as well. Additionally, in the EU, EMA also provides a formal framework for regular interaction with the industry through various channels, including provision of scientific advice to companies involved in research and development, oversight of the centralised procedures and special guidance to SMEs. Such support and guidance is provided with the aim of increasing compliance and facilitating clarity in interpreting complex rules and regulations. Similarly, USFDA and Japan's Pharmaceutical and Medical Devices Agency (PMDA) have regulatory frameworks that contain a structured and formal system for industry and regulatory agency interactions.

Harmonisation has been considered an advantage for the MNCs and export oriented companies due to their easy access to markets that follow common global standards. This has been particularly true in the case of Singapore where the industry has benefited on two accounts : 1) the large base of MNCs versus a much smaller local industry, 2) HSA's acceptance of the ICH CTD, standardised guidelines and its participation in collaboration initiatives. But it is also important to assess its impact on the local and small scale companies as well. It is often argued that implementation of global standards through harmonisation may create a barrier for local companies and lead to unnecessary increase in regulatory requirements (Lezotre 2014).[6] Along with the high standards that would have to be followed by these local companies, it would also attract more foreign companies. This has been reflected in some of the ASEAN countries as there is a concern among the SMEs about increased competition from the integrated ASEAN healthcare sector. Implementation of GMP guidelines is particularly a matter of concern for them as it may drive them out of business.[7] This was corroborated during the field interactions that the Indonesian generic producing local companies for this reason have been resistant towards harmonisation until now. But the respondents also expressed that lately these companies have foreseen a benefit as harmonisation would open the gates to international markets and increase their export capabilities. Currently they mainly cater to domestic needs of the country.

The impact on local companies may have far reaching public health implications in developing countries. WHO (2001) highlighted the fact that in many countries, essential drugs required for the prevention and treatment of locally endemic conditions are not supplied by the major multinationals, but by local industry or the generic manufacturers. Thus, if these companies are unable to meet the higher standardised guidelines (like that of ICH), it may lead to withdrawal of these drugs which will adversely impact public health. This does not suggest that companies should continue working on lower standards but should attain at least the desirable minimum at the earliest. Following on, with government support and sufficient time given, companies will be able to achieve higher standards so that public health is not compromised in any way.

Interestingly, in contrast to the concerns mentioned, no resistance has been shown by the industry in South Africa.[8] In fact , they have seen an

6. Lezotre considers this concern as legitimate because in order to harmonize a topic between countries, it may lead to combining of all current requirements from different countries (i.e., if one country requests Study A and another country requests Study B for the registration of new medicines, a quick solution would be to ask for both Studies A and B) which will be unreasonable and should be carefully dealt with.

7. See *http://pdf.usaid.gov/pdf_docs/Pnadj869.pdf* (Last accessed on 15 April 2017).

8. In fact, particularly in the SADC region, the initial guidelines were developed in consultation with the industry but were taken over by regulators after sometime. During our field interactions, we learnt that industry once again seems to be coming back in a more proactive role, recognising the critical imperative harmonisation would serve to boost trade within the region.

immediate advantage for the local pharmaceutical manufacturers as it will provide them with easier access to markets in the larger Sub-Saharan African region. This is especially important since some of the smaller countries in the larger African region are otherwise very small, seemingly non-viable markets, which in the absence of harmonisation, may not provide enough incentive to firms to supply their products there. That is also one of the benefits that will come out of having joint assessments procedures such as ZAZIBONA in the African region and PAN-ASEAN registration and SIAHR that is in discussions among ASEAN member states. Similarly, in the US, the generic drug industry has agreed to most provisions of the ICH but it seeks to have more participation than it has right now. Industry experts believe that through opportunities for participation, they can address some of the issues that differ in the level of detail. The generic drug industry is also in favour of more mutual recognition programmes that will allow exchange of information and enable sharing of scarce resources. This seems to be particularly important for overseas inspections which can be quite costly to carry out. The interviewees also expressed that generic players anticipate that greater harmonisation will reduce the currently high fluctuations in prices within the US. However, this would be feasible only if the bar (for standards) is set appropriately such that every player, regardless of the scale of operation, can comply with these standards.

A predominant view that emerged from our field interactions suggested that while pathways like harmonisation of various regulatory requirements often entails high costs for the smaller players, the benefits would exceed costs over time with adequate support mechanisms from the government. For instance, Europe provides a viable solution through the Office of SMEs at the EMA which facilitates scientific advice and technical guidance at a lower fee, to mitigate the cost associated with centralised procedure, and to promote innovation and development of new products by SMEs.[9] Further, the EMA also provides early and proactive support to medicine developers in order to enhance and enable accelerated assessment of medicine applications under the PRIME scheme.

Having discussed various aspects of international cooperation, it is important to acknowledge its impact on industry and hence, public health. Accordingly, our way forward in the direction of international cooperation should take due cognizance of our country's unique characteristics and requirements. A country's internal concerns such as those for the SMEs operating within its jurisdiction are genuine and can be addressed through government support at various stages. This could be addressed through regular interactions between industry and regulator, which can lead to formation and enforcement of functional and practical guidelines hence striving for more efficient regulatory processes.

9. See: Commission Regulation (EC) No 2049/2005, retrieved from *http://eur-lex.europa.eu/LexUriServ/LexUriServ.do?uri=OJ:L:2005:329:0004:0007:EN:PDF* (Last accessed on 14 February 2017). Also, equally facilitating are programmes like Horizon 2020 programme, which aims at augmenting research and development in EU. Such programmes offer support at different stages—some programmes only fund early development—startup phase, follow-on phase, but it is changing since couple of year with some new measures that also fund clinical development—early stages: phase 1 and phase 2.

5

A Game Theoretic Approach to Understanding International Cooperation

Consider the following model with two countries, A and B. Each has the choice to either to switch its standards/guidelines/protocols and reap the benefits from cooperation and coordination, or to remain status quo. In order to understand international cooperation as a coordination game, we borrow the following model from Drezner (2005) and extend it by bringing in variation in adjustment costs for the two players. Given that there are significant differences between domestic regulatory protocols of the countries to begin with, there would be certain costs involved in making any changes to the status quo, which may be political and administrative in nature. On the other hand, not cooperating with each other and retaining status quo, may also prove costly for countries since they would lose out on the potential benefits of cooperation.

Figure 5.1

Payoff Matrix

		Country B	
		Switch	Do not switch
Country A	Switch	$-d_A, -d_B$	$\pi_A - d_A, \pi_B$
	Do not switch	$\pi_A - \pi_B, d_B$	$-c_A, -c_B$

Here (see Figure 5.1) π_i is the benefit to country from cooperating with the other country.

d_i is the cost of adjustment incurred by country i if it opts to participate in international cooperation initiatives.

c_i is the cost to be borne by country i if it chooses to retain status quo.

We first assume here that the benefits from cooperation are more than the costs of adjustment i.e. $\pi_i > d_i$.

The best responses of the players then are as follows:

- The best response for country A when country B decides to switch is to not switch.
- The best response for country A when country B decides to not to switch is to switch.
- The best response for country B when country A decides to switch is not to switch.
- The best response for country B when country A decides to not to switch is to switch.

This results in the following two equilibria (switch, do not switch) and (do not switch, switch). Both of these are cooperating equilibria however, in order to establish which one is superior to the other we have to take into consideration the market size and market power of the two countries. In order to do so, we consider the following 3 scenarios.

Scenario 1:

If country B has more stringent guidelines/protocols, then it will be beneficial for country A to adopt B's guidelines/protocols rather than the other way around. Moving to more stringent guidelines/protocols among the two countries will result in welfare enhancement for both players. If we consider this scenario, then the superior equilibrium among the two is when country A switches and country B chooses not to switch.

Scenario 2:

If country A has more stringent guidelines/protocols to begin with then the outcome will be the same as above except that now it is in the interest of country B to adopt country A's guidelines/protocols. So, the superior equilibrium is (do not switch, switch).

Scenario 3:

In this case, consider both are at par to begin with or that the benefits to cooperation and coordination are rather similar. Then both the equilibria would be equivalent.

In the instance when we are considering international cooperation on pharmaceutical standards, registration procedures etc., scenario 1 and 2 above would aptly represent the situation of two players with widely different protocols. Hence, if a developing country considers upward integration, then it would result in a superior welfare outcome since there would be public health as well as trade related benefits, due to an ease of access to quality medicines. This situation could also be modelled around a different set of players: a developing country such as India and an existing harmonisation/cooperation initiative such as the ICH/IGDRP/ASEAN. Here again, it would be optimal for a developing country to adopt protocols of a cooperation initiative which are modelled around those of a mature regulatory jurisdiction. For instance, the current operating environment in India allows existence of dual standards for drugs, i.e., one standard for the domestic market and relatively higher standards for export markets. This situation, if allowed to prevail, might lead to a scenario where lower standards become a regular occurrence, given that there is pre-existing information asymmetry associated with pharmaceutical products. While it should be noted that varying pharmacopeal standards across the world are a common phenomenon and not an issue unique to India, we wish to draw attention to the fact that for India the gap between the internal and the minimum international standards is quite significant. More importantly, further stringent regulatory protocols, in general, are in favour of improved public health. As mentioned earlier, using 'anti-lemon devices' such as policies aimed at streamlining the regulatory environment and uplifting existing standards, will contribute towards weeding out manufacturers of fake or substandard medicines and this will help in providing the much needed credibility in terms of quality. Hence, an effort needs to be made to ensure internal harmonisation,[1] which will be a stepping stone in the direction of achieving higher standards of public health, global competitiveness, and greater confidence in the health system, and more meaningful opportunities for international cooperation.

The costs of switching guidelines/protocols here can be envisioned as the costs to various players within the pharmaceutical sector. The technical costs to the government/regulator will be that of administering new protocols, through increasing the regulatory bandwidth in terms of human, financial and technological resources. On the other hand, costs to the industry will vary across segments of the industry, being relatively less for the larger players who may already be complying with more stringent guidelines/protocols for their export market. The costs are likely to be significant for medium and small players who have a limited scale of production and/or might export to countries with relatively less stringent requirements and protocols. However, those small players who are neither engaged in manufacturing of new drugs nor are export oriented, but manufacture drugs that are no longer new (for which more than 4 years have elapsed since their first approval) for the local market, are also likely to face significant adjustment costs if the domestic procedures become more streamlined with those at the international level.

It may be noted that adjustment to more stringent guidelines and protocols is possible without compromising national sovereignty and should be seen as a way to strengthen national regulatory resources. In this regard, as highlighted before, convergence has emerged as a popular pathway of international cooperation.

The proposition for upward integration, however, is not without its own set of limitations. While moving towards international protocols might result in a superior welfare outcome, there arises some measure of concern regarding small-scale companies, which are faced with challenges in relation to their costs and the technical expertise required in adopting such guidelines. Thus, it is recommended that such companies be given a longer time frame to implement the new guidelines and should receive initial support from the government.

Consider the example of moving towards eCTD, which would require all players—regardless of their size—to switch to e-submission in the prescribed format. This has benefits, as elucidated earlier in this report, for the regulator (faster and more efficient reviews) and for the manufacturer (less expensive to produce the dossier and savings in shipping costs). However, the smaller industry players without adequate wherewithals to switch from paper based to e-submission, will be faced with significant challenges to begin with. Nevertheless, having a common protocol across manufacturers is certainly more efficient (with support provided to smaller industry players in the initial stages) than the current system that allows variations.

1. It has been pointed out earlier that in addition to the role of the central regulator, the day-to-day implementation and monitoring of the DCA is the responsibility of the state drug regulatory authorities. However, there are often differences that can be found in the actual implementation across states. Thus, it is recommended that an effort towards internal harmonisation be made to reduce these differences and have a uniform set of standards across the country.

6

Policy Recommendations

The current section presents policy recommendations which have been drawn up keeping in mind various challenges faced by Indian stakeholders identified in earlier sections. Further, these are reflective of the experience and best practices from selected jurisdictions in tackling similar challenges. This would be one of the first attempts at documenting a more priority based systemic approach to address international cooperation in the realm of medicine registration in India.

The foremost step in this direction would be to set a time bound and targeted vision for pharmaceutical regulations. Therefore, every recommendation is provided with a feasible time frame, such as, short (six months to one year), medium (one to three years) and long term (more than three years). Each recommendation is targeted at various relevant departments of the government given the role of each in the process of pharmaceutical regulation.

In order to reap maximum benefits from various international cooperation initiatives, the system of drug regulation in India will need to overcome structural, procedural and legislative challenges. The ongoing effort to revisit the DCA is expected to give some impetus to this process.[1] Further, recommendations and the way they can be operationalised are highlighted below along with a plausible time frame to achieve the goal.

6.1 International Cooperation

A. Periodic Assessment of New Drug Approvals

To identify areas of unmet medical needs which the regulator can address by engaging in various international cooperation initiatives

Time Frame

Medium-term/Long-term.

Operationalisation

India's participation in international cooperation initiatives should be based on their relevance to India's challenges. Further, collaborations should be encouraged in the spirit of active participation of all stakeholders (agency, industry, civil society) towards contributing to global collaborative efforts of streamlining medicine regulation, including scientific areas that are most meaningful to India's environment. The Indian regulator, whose mandate is to both protect and promote public health, by carrying out periodic assessments of drug approvals (may be on an annual basis), can identify the areas of under-served medical needs. Subsequently, the government can consider providing expedited review pathways for such disease categories, may be through international agreements like CECA that Singapore has in place for faster entry of India made generics into its domestic market. By providing incentives to companies, the regulator can ensure that it meets its public health goals by bringing in newer treatment options.

Potential challenges that may arise in operationalising the recommendation

It should be recognised that international cooperation initiatives, alone will not guarantee drug development in all areas of unmet medical needs in our country. This is partly because neglected diseases or diseases that are not prevalent globally but are prevalent in India or other populations, are often not on the agenda for global pharmaceutical companies. Therefore, insofar as expediting the drug approval process is concerned, international cooperation initiatives are a means towards this end and should not be viewed as the end in itself.

It may be noted that all DRAs face a continuous dichotomy of faster medicine approval as well as ensuring access to safe medicines. While additional tests and documentation act as effective checks and balances to minimise potential risk associated with the medicine, it may delay access to crucial medicines (Philipson and Sun 2010: 3).[2] Efficient medicine registration process, thus, is one of the most critical factors in ensuring availability and access to safe medicine. Keeping this in mind, mature jurisdictions including USFDA and EMA provide certain FRPs (facilitated regulatory pathways)[3] at every stage of

1. See Notice dated 6 June 2016 by CDSCO: *http://www.cdsco.nic.in/writereaddata/Noticedatede06_6_2016.pdf* (Last accessed on 15 April 2017).

2. Literature suggests, this dichotomy can pose potential decision-making challenges for the regulator which can have paradoxical outcomes: 'Type 1 error': approving a drug which proves to be unsafe and lesser effective; and 'Type 2 error': delaying approval of otherwise acceptable and safe medicine (Carpenter 2004, Puig-Junoy 2005, Copland and Howard 2009 and Philipson and Sun 2010).

3. As discussed in the previous sections, in US FDA, there are provisions in form of priority review, accelerated assessment, breakthrough therapy, fast track, orphan drug status; whereas in EMA facilitates provisions like adaptive pathways, PRIME, conditional marketing authorisation, granting of marketing authorisation under exceptional circumstances, and orphan drug status to the drug. These routes are offered by the said jurisdictions with iterative process of scientific advice and guidance beginning from the early stages of drug development.

drug development, if the applicant can prove that the medicine demonstrates substantial gains to existing line of treatment or caters to an unmet medical need.

At present, there are no formal FRPs offered by the Indian regulator. However, recent developments in the regulatory space have provided some impetus towards prioritising registration of certain medicines in the country. First, as per the order of the Supreme Court, the MoHFW[4] has made it mandatory for all the applicants of GCTs/NCEs to provide information on assessment of risk versus benefit to the patients, innovation vis-à-vis existing therapeutic option, and unmet medical need in the country. Second, in terms of expediting the review of certain essential drugs, the Apex Committee has recommended that for drugs already approved outside India, waiver of CT in Indian population may be considered only in cases of national emergency, extreme urgency, epidemic and for orphan drugs for rare diseases and drugs indicated for conditions/diseases for which there is no therapy.[5] In furtherance to this, the consideration for CT waivers are decided by the Apex Committee on the recommendation of SEC and Technical Committee, on a case by case basis, reflections of which are published in the minutes of the meeting of the various committees. These developments are indicative of the regulatory thinking, however, substantive regulatory guidance is required insofar as the exact definition and requirements to be presented for unmet medical needs are concerned. Bhat (2015) and Sangai et al. (2016) have laid down a range of challenges in the prioritisation of medicines—including lack of clarity in definition of unmet medical need and concomitant rationale to grant waivers for conducting CTs—despite having the three tier (expert committees) review mechanism in place.

Hence decoding the meaning of *unmet medical needs* would be challenging for the regulator given the lack of adequate variables and data to define it. This would be particularly difficult with the complexity associated with 'access' to treatment in India, which is two pronged—lack of access to available treatment options and lack of access to newer treatment options. Further, weak disease surveillance mechanisms make it difficult to attribute the real areas of unmet medical needs as a rare disease indication may not be reflected in the existing data on disease burden.

Given the absence of adequate formal guidance, such as that on the lines of orphan drug legislation, defining critical terms like 'rare diseases'[6], 'unmet medical needs' is imperative for bringing clarity on regulatory expectations. In the absence of such regulatory provisions, prioritising medicine registration, and associated benefits from international cooperation would continue to be a challenging task for the regulator.

> *B. Learning Opportunities at Global Forums*
>
> India should seek learning opportunities at global forums such as ICH and IGDRP.

Time Frame

Medium-term.

Operationalisation

As an initial step, participating in meetings of global forums will benefit India as it can learn from the experiences of mature regulatory jurisdictions and become a part of the expert discussions. Thus opportunities like observership at forums such as that of the ICH will help India in gaining insights, putting across its own concerns, adopting best practices and bringing about feasible changes domestically as well.

Additionally, such forums have already worked on and established scientific guidelines that can be considered for adoption by India. Hence, these learning opportunities can help India build its policies based on its own national framework, instead of reinventing the wheel.

> *C. Regional Cooperation Initiatives*
>
> India could explore potential cooperation initiatives (likes of ZAZIBONA, EU) with countries that have similar disease burdens.

4. See Order of DCGI dated 5 September 2014: *http://www.cdsco.nic.in/writereaddata/office%20order%20dated%2005_09_2014.pdf* (Last accessed on 15 February 2017).
5. See the Minutes of the APEX committee meeting held on 27 February 2015: *http://cdsco.nic.in/writereaddata/21st%20-%20Apex-%20Minutes%20of%20meeting.pdf* (Last accessed on 15 February 2017).
6. Discussions around the need for a national policy on rare diseases, and orphan drug legislation, have gained momentum in the policy circles. The most recent one being a discussion meeting on policy framework associated with 'rare diseases', organised on 23 February 2017 at Jawaharlal Nehru University, New Delhi.

Time Frame

Long-term.

Operationalisation

In order to address some of the concerns that emerged during field interactions with respect to duplication of efforts involved in review of applications, and lack of technical expertise with the regulator leading to additional challenges; joint assessments with the experts of mature jurisdictions can be explored as an alternate pathway (a joint review collaboration with neighbouring countries or with countries with similar disease burden or pharmerging economies like BRICS). Such collaborations are being followed by some African countries as well as countries in Europe, and is expected to enhance reviewing capabilities, which will facilitate faster introduction of safe, good quality, and efficacious drugs. Additionally, collaborations and learning from the assessment reports of other countries will be of immense value, especially in the case of novel drugs that have the potential to address unmet medical needs.

There is much to gain from joint assessments among countries that share a similar pattern of disease burden. The diseases prevalent in developing countries at times may differ from the ones in the western world. Thus, to address the specific requirements in their countries, developing nations can come together and focus on a collective approval process of drugs that address local needs. In addition to this, these countries can together participate in FRPs through international cooperation programmes and thus receive guidance from the experts of mature jurisdictions such as the US and the EU. Examples include, Article 58 of the EMA,[7] which aims at increasing access to drugs in low and middle income countries (LMICs). Similar to this is the FDA procedure called PEPFAR,[8] which facilitates generic drug registration in low income countries and has helped in capacity building in sub-Saharan African region. PEPFAR focuses on a transition from emergency response to an epidemic, to sustainable country programmes and enables such responses to be country owned and country driven. Hence, it supports countries in taking leadership of the responses to their epidemics and is increasing collaboration with multilateral organisations.[9] These examples highlight the role regional cooperation can play in addressing public health goals.

The issue of neglected diseases (diseases that are not prevalent globally but are prevalent particularly in India or other populations), highlighted in the recommendation above, maybe addressed through a regional cooperation initiative as well. Thus, if a regional group is formed on the basis of similar disease patterns/epidemics and have collective demand for medicines for those diseases, then it can act as an incentive for the companies due to the availability of potential market. Companies will find it further enticing if collective registration of medicines (common document such as ACTD and a collective review) is provided in this regional block so that drug approval becomes easy. Hence, the countries will benefit from the timely availability of necessary drugs and companies will gain from easy application processes and the availability of a ready market.

Furthermore, such regional initiatives can collaborate among themselves and form larger cooperation blocks. This will help in bringing more economies together and ensure an enhanced sharing of information and expertise. A recent example of a regional block (although not in the health or the pharmaceutical sector) that has been successful is the BRICS-BIMSTEC[10] engagement, India being the common member to both.[11] This regional block

7. As explained before, Article 58 of Regulation (EC) No 726/2004, introduced first in 2004, allows EMA's CHMP in cooperation with the World Health Organization (WHO), to give opinions on drugs which are intended exclusively for markets outside the EU to prevent or treat diseases of major public health interest.

8. The US President's Emergency Plan for AIDS Relief (PEPFAR) is a US Government initiative to help save the lives the people suffering from HIV/AIDS around the world. It also helps alleviate suffering from other diseases. It is driven by a shared responsibility among donor and partner nations and others to make smart investments to save lives

9. For details, see *http://www.pepfar.gov/about/* (Last accessed on 10 April 2017).

10. BRICS is the acronym for an association of five major emerging national economies: Brazil, Russia, India, China and South Africa, all leading developing or newly industrialised countries.
The Bay of Bengal Initiative for Multi-Sectoral Technical and Economic Cooperation (BIMSTEC) is an international organisation involving a group of countries in South Asia and South East Asia. These are: Bangladesh, India, Myanmar, Sri Lanka, Thailand, Bhutan and Nepal. It is a technological and economic cooperation among South Asian and Southeast Asian countries along the coast of the Bay of Bengal

11. For instance: The 6th BRICS Health Ministers Meeting in India included discussion and adoption of action plans on specific areas of cooperation areas among the BRICS countries in the realm of health care. Focus areas include strengthening regulatory systems in case of international and national health emergencies, collaboration towards promotion of research and development of innovative medical products

contd...

cooperates on common objectives as well as learns from the achievements each has made in different areas and thus complements each other.[12] Drawing insights from such an economic integration, regional initiatives (existing or the ones likely to be formed in future) in the field of drug registrations and the pharmaceutical sector can have global impacts through their associations with each other and eventually develop larger networks that will result in reducing duplication of efforts, increasing access to medicines and addressing urgent medical needs, a concern in most of the developing nations as of today. Ongoing efforts being made in this direction are reflected in that of ASEAN, which is an observer at the ICH and draws upon its guidelines from the forum, if they find them locally suitable and applicable. Regional cooperation can be beneficial even if under-resourced regulators collaborate, as has been done in ZAZIBONA.

Potential challenges that may arise in operationalising the recommendation

Regional initiatives face challenges due to the varied local characteristics of its member countries, which can make it difficult for every country to agree with all decisions. ASEAN is a case in point here; the impact of harmonisation has been different among its member states due to their background, local industry conditions, level of economic development, regulatory requirements and capacities etc. Further, differences in the willingness to harmonise, lack of trust and political relations between economies may result in varying outcomes. A BRICS-BIMSTEC type of engagement might be challenging in the field of medicine for the same reasons, but such partnerships among groups can strive to achieve harmonisation in the registration of medicines; given the common public health objectives. It might also take time consuming research efforts to establish areas of neglected diseases and accordingly form a regional block.

6.2 Drug Registration Procedures: Dossier Submission and Review

A. Pre-filing Consultation for an Efficient Registration Process

Time Frame

Medium-term.

Operationalisation

In order to make sure that the most efficient process of drug registration and approval is followed, regulators in a number of international jurisdictions have provisions for a pre-submission consultation. Such meetings,when facilitated at the IND stage, could provide agency's advice on the studies required for making a successful application. Further,such consultations prior to submission of NDA gives an opportunity for the regulator and the applicant to sit together and discuss the necessary data and documentation that would be required during the approval process. Having these initial meetings greatly reduces the chances of delays in the approval process because of incomplete documentation or lack of clarity of regulators' expectations. Improving the quality of the dossier submitted reduces the need to raise queries during the approval cycle. Thus, with this consultation, a smoother and more efficient registration process is expected to follow.

In India, as of now, each dossier is examined at the time of submission for completeness by nodal officers appointed at the CDSCO. This is purely an administrative check, which only examines the documents submitted as per a checklist and there is no thorough consultation through which the applicant can ensure compliance with all regulatory requirements.[13] Therefore, while an administrative review helps in identifying gaps in documentation, as a precursor, pre-submission consultations between the regulator and the applicant will greatly ease the process as a whole and improve the quality of dossiers submitted.

...contd...

(drugs, vaccines and medical technologies), promotion of existing IT platform and regulatory capacity building through an institutional development plan for BRICS countries, joint efforts towards tackling communicable and non-communicable disease, development and production of quality-assured drugs, diagnostics and vaccines.

12. Such as in this collaboration, BRICS is expected to benefit by studying the progress achieved by BIMSTEC in certain fields including counter terrorism while BIMSTEC can benefit from the experience and expertise of large economies of BRICS in infrastructure and connectivity building or energy.

13. Provision to introduce pre-submission meetings was proposed vide CDSCO's Notice dated 28 January 2015. However, as on date, no formal guidance is available regarding the same. See: *http://www.cdsco.nic.in/writereaddata/NOTICE15.pdf* (Last accessed on 15 April 2017).

Potential challenges that may arise in operationalising the recommendation

The medicine regulator could face two apparent challenges in implementing the aforementioned recommendation. First, there is the concern that, at present, the CDSCO does not have enough experts to conduct such a pre-filing consultation. As of now, there are just 18 senior experts at the regulators' office, including the Drugs Controller General, Joint Drugs Controllers, Deputy Drugs Controllers, and Assistant Drugs Controllers and 132 inspectors. Compared with the numerous responsibilities that they are entrusted with, the CDSCO will certainly need more hands to start pre-filing consultations. There may also be a need to carefully evaluate whether pre-filing consultations will be required for every category of a NDA.

A second concern relates to the nature of the advice —whether and to what extent the advice would be binding upon the agency. This is particularly important in scenarios wherein due to changes in the rules or regulatory expectations, CDSCO could request additional data or deviate from the guidance provided in the initial consultation.

B. Procedural Clarity

Extensive guidance documents explaining the process, timelines and requirements for a marketing authorisation application to bring about procedural clarity.

Time Frame

Short-term/Medium-term.

Operationalisation

Guidance documents that outline regulatory expectations are useful supplements to legislations. India has recently released a detailed document explaining the marketing authorisation requirements for biosimilars.[14] It would be helpful to have similar documents, i.e., substantive guidelines on the studies required for approval and procedural guidelines, for all the NDAs specifying the details of various regulatory requirements, timelines, and conditions for CT/biowaivers, etc.

Over and above checklists of documents, which are listed on the CDSCO website, such guidance documents can be linked to *SUGAM information portal* in order to ensure real time dissemination of information. This could lead to significant saving of resources, both regulatory and that of the industry, as in many cases, online availability of relevant guidance could reduce the time taken to contact a nodal regulatory official. Additionally, the regulator can also provide a list of frequently asked questions on the *SUGAM information portal*. As regulation is a dynamic process, there is a definite need for periodic revision of such guidance documents to reflect the policy changes. Given that the regulator is considering remodelling the regulatory process to a paperless and an electronic one, information through the SUGAM portal would also aid the ad hoc information dissemination and build an institutional memory. This would help the regulator in organising, identifying and better addressing the regulatory gaps.

Furthermore, linking all the SDRAs with *SUGAM information portal* will create a common information platform, as well as help tackle the perennial issue of lack of uniformity in the interpretation of regulatory procedures among CDSCO and SDRAs.

Potential challenges that may arise in operationalising the recommendation

First and the foremost challenge is the time and resources required to prepare exhaustive, substantive and procedural guidance documents. Since the guidance documents reflect regulatory expectations, they should be prepared keeping in mind the existing challenges faced by various stakeholders. Hence, proactive engagement of stakeholders while formulating such documents could be extremely beneficial for compliance. Agencies like US FDA and EMA make their expectations quite clear in the guidance documents and most of those in the industry understand and act accordingly when complying with various regulations.

Second, linking all the SDRAs will be a challenge, given the current lack of the requisite infrastructural wherewithal. Nevertheless, in this direction there are deliberations[15] about linking the SUGAM portal with the XLN software. This recommendation will, therefore, require dedicated workforce for

14. See: Guidelines on Similar Biologics: Regulatory Requirements for Marketing Authorisation in India. Retrieved from: *http://www.cdsco.nic.in/writereaddata/Bio%20Similar%20Guideline.pdf* (Last accessed on 30 January 2017).

15. Information as provided in the 50th Drugs Consultative Committee meeting held on 4 and 5 November 2016. Please see: *http://cdsco.nic.in/writereaddata/ddc50report.pdf* (Last accessed on 15 February 2017).

maintaining and updating the *SUGAM information portal* on a day-to-day basis.

C. Life Cycle Approach to the Dossier Format and Submission Process

Bridging the gap between SUGAM and the internationally followed eCTD (electronic common technical document) to provide a life cycle approach to the dossier format and submission process.

Time Frame

Long-term.

Operationalisation

It has been highlighted earlier that SUGAM is being seen as a game changer in the realm of drug regulation in India. However, firms operating on a global scale are already reaping the benefits of eCTD as a submission gateway, which is no longer confined to the ICH member countries. Regulators in several jurisdictions have found it useful to adopt and adapt eCTD within their systems since it offers a unique and efficient mechanism for submission as well as review of applications. In the present scenario, when it seems like most countries are tending towards a common platform, India might also consider adapting the same. This could be done by bridging the gap between the presently existing SUGAM platform, which is only a submission platform, to the eCTD format which has a dual gateway and will facilitate greater information sharing/exchange between various global regulatory partners.[16]

Some recent developments on the block, include the proposal of the health ministry to extend the validity of a new drug from a period of 4 years to 10 years.[17] If such a move materialises, then every subsequent applicant of an already approved molecule will approach the CDSCO for another 6 years, which as per the present rules is taken care of by the SDRAs. This will greatly increase the quantum of work at the CDCSO, which will require more manpower. In an alternate scenario, if the current four-year rule is entirely done away with, it would also increase the quantum of applications that the CDSCO receives. Even in the case, status quo prevails, the regulator should give consideration to adopting an increasingly streamlined protocol that would immensely enhance the efficiency of the process.

Potential challenges that may arise in operationalising the recommendation

There may be practical challenges in achieving this, given that SUGAM is already operational and significant costs have been invested in setting up the system.

When SUGAM is transformed into eCTD, it will work as a sender-receiver model. This implies that once the applicant submits the dossier through the platform, not only the regulator but the reviewer will also have online access to the dossier. Through the new software, the reviewers will be able to examine the application and add their comments on it. As per the present system, only the CDCSO staff have access to the SUGAM software, and bridging the gap between the SUGAM portal and the eCTD may result in additional hurdles because then every reviewer's system will have to be fitted with the new software. This implies further training costs as well. While not entirely impossible, such a change will raise technical difficulties initially and will generate significant costs for the exchequer.

D. In-house Reviewers

Building in a team of in-house reviewers to create institutional memory.

Time Frame

Medium-term/Long-term.

Operationalisation

At present, the review of a new drug application undergoes a three-tier sequential process, involving the SEC/IND committees, Technical Committee, and Apex Committee.

The said system was devised by MoHFW to strengthen the review process and in compliance with a Supreme Court's order[18] regarding supervision

16. A mapping exercise of content differences between SUGAM and the eCTD would have been beneficial, however, given SUGAM portal and eCTD are evolving on a continuous basis, it would not be feasible to do so.

17. Information as provided in the Minutes of the 74th Meeting of Drugs Technical Advisory Board held on 15 November 2016 at DGHS: *http://www.cdsco.nic.in/writereaddata/MOM%2074th%20DTAB.pdf* (Last accessed on 15 February 2017).

18. Order dated 3 January 2013, in the matter of W.P. (C) No. 33/2012 of Swasthya Adhikar Manch, Indore & Anr Vs. Ministry of Health and Family Welfare & Ors. with WP(C) No. 779/2012.

of clinical trial applications. However, as highlighted before, the three-tier sequential review process is reported to be cumbersome and complicated. This is primarily because the regulator critically relies on a set of external reviewers, who are experts in their respective fields, and are involved full-time at the primary institution to which they are affiliated. For every application that comes in to the CDSCO, a committee of reviewers is decided upon and they are periodically called in for meetings during which they evaluate the dossier through its various stages. This is not an easy process since the regulators' office has to expend considerable time in order to coordinate between these experts, as some of them are based at various places across the country. In addition, it is also a costly exercise since the regulator has to bear the cost of calling in these experts repeatedly for meetings. Besides, once these applications are finalised, at times there is no institutional memory created as to how the approval process takes place. In addition to in-house experts, MoHFW can have the opinion of the said committees on a need/case-to-case basis. Even in other jurisdictions, there are in-house review experts, over and above the specialised committees which may be consulted for additional inputs.

In the light of what has been said before, having in-house reviewers will not only be more time as well as cost efficient, but will strengthen the institutional memory and create a team of experts who are solely dedicated to this task. As a supplementary measure and a long term goal, it would be imperative for the government to strengthen the ecosystem facilitating specialised education in regulatory sciences. Such specialists could be directly recruited into the regulatory system thereby making dossier review a primary responsibility for them.

Potential challenges that may arise in operationalising the recommendation

Building an in-house review team is a time and resource intensive process. The regulator will need to plan the composition of the review team, required budget, and targeted timeline to implement this. This would be critical given the ongoing reform measures to revamp the existing DCA and deliberations in the government forums regarding introduction of a new drug policy. As discussed before, changes bearing an impact on the existing 'new drug' (4 year new drug status) definition in Rule 122E of DCR, would also affect the medicine registration process and associated regulatory workload of CDSCO. This could potentially affect the number of subsequent NDAs to the CDSCO.

Additionally, in order to avoid uncertainties, adequate guidance to communicate the changes to various stakeholders will be required. Since regulatory procedures are extremely dynamic, periodic training modules and sessions for the reviewers will be required to keep them abreast of the latest regulatory science technologies and best practices.

> *E. Working of Review Project Managers*
>
> Review project managers to work in tandem with the review experts, to ensure timeliness in the review process.

Time Frame

Medium-term.

Operationalisation

In order to facilitate a lifecycle approach to medicine approvals, including project managers in addition to in-house reviewers will help CDSCO ensure a time-bound review process. The project managers will also act as a nodal point for a smooth interface between the regulator and the applicant. In several jurisdictions, this has helped in ensuring that the review is completed within the scheduled timeline and enhanced the level of transparency and accountability in the regulatory approval process.

Potential Challenges that May Arise in Operationalising the Recommendation

Since review project managers will facilitate a lifecycle approach to drug approval process, it will be imperative for the regulator to assess the number of such personnel required with the quantum of applications. This could be assessed based on the nature and type of applications that are received by CDSCO. There will also be a need to clearly specify the nature of their work,which in turn, would be based on the budgetary flexibilities of the regulatory authority.

6.3 Addressing Additional Gaps

> *A. Collate a Dataset*
>
> A comprehensive dataset can be collated through SUGAM, which further can be useful to conduct regulatory impact assessments.

Time Frame

Medium-term.

Operationalisation

In order to operationalise this recommendation, CDCSO will have to further broaden the ambit of SUGAM on a much wider scale. The SUGAM portal can be used to compile such a dataset with details on applications and approvals by type of drug, time to approval, etc. A rich dataset that is publicly accessible will enable researchers to carry out an effective analysis of the various regulatory policies of the government. By conducting a natural experiment,[19] it will allow one to see whether a certain policy has had the desired effect or not. This will go a long way in helping design better policies by addressing gaps in previous policies and ensuring better implementation of existing policies.

Potential challenges that may arise in operationalising the recommendation

The major challenge here can be with respect to the significant costs to be incurred by the regulator in building this dataset. There would be also be a need to appoint some personnel on a full-time basis to monitor the databank and update it real-time. Thus, there will be both administrative and technical costs involved in implementing this recommendation.

B. Focus on Internal Harmonisation

India must focus on internal harmonisation (streamlining the processes domestically, aiming at uniform implementation of DCA across states) and provide the support for small scale industry that will be needed during this process.

Time Frame

Long-term.

Operationalisation

Given the presence of a huge and vibrant pharmaceutical industry in India, one of the critical factors required for a smooth functioning regulatory environment is uniform implementation of rules and guidelines. In India, manufacturing hubs are located at various places across the country which are directly regulated by the local state authorities. The problem arises when there are differences in the implementation of the rules and guidelines across states. Once there is renewed focus on internal harmonisation, it will require manufacturers across the country to be on equal footing with respect to regulatory protocols. An added benefit to this will enable reducing the gap between the current domestic standards and those being met for the export markets.

Potential challenges that may arise in operationalising the recommendation

The above said recommendation could have twofold challenges which need to be duly addressed. First, there would be need for significant investment of time and other resources for bringing about a transition in the DRAs across the countries which at the present have varying regulatory capacities. Second, given that this transition may not be easy for the smaller industry players there would be need for providing them with planned and dedicated support in the initial stages.

19. Natural experiments are studies in which there is a transparent exogenous source of variation in the explanatory variables that determine the treatment assignment. A natural experiment induced by policy changes, government randomisation, or other events may allow a researcher to obtain exogenous variation in the main explanatory variables (Meyer 1995).

7

Conclusion

Given 'unnecessary differences' in local regulatory procedures for drug registration combined with differential local regulatory capacities, the cross border movement—and universal availability—of medicines is not as seamless as one would hope, to say the least. Several national regulators have come together to cooperate and address the challenges of public health and facilitate ease of doing business for pharmaceutical industry—ICH, ASEAN, AMRH and IGDRP being some examples.

Improved and more efficient drug registration processes are critical not only in the backdrop of the changing dynamics of the Indian pharmaceutical industry and its efforts towards drug discovery, but, more importantly, in the wake of the rapidly changing burden of disease and demand for newer and better treatment options in the country. Nevertheless, Indian drug regulators have largely stayed away from ongoing initiatives of international cooperation, despite India being a signatory to the international health goals—earlier under the MDG, and now the SDG, framework of the United Nations—as well as growing international participation and stature of the country generally. Indian regulatory framework cannot operate in isolation from the general aspiration and approach of the Government of India as far as external affairs and international participation are concerned, not to talk of India's critical need to tackle its health challenges, particularly the massive burden of premature mortality (see Mehdi et al. 2016).

In the preceding pages, we have discussed issues with respect to drug registration within India, the ways in which international cooperation has helped address similar issues in other jurisdictions and developed specific policy recommendations. In order to maximise benefits from international cooperation in the realm of registration of medicines, there is a need to streamline related processes as a precursor to having meaningful cooperation. As the first and foremost step, India has to address domestic issues—both structural and legislative—and provide a strong foundation for effective regulation. Having transparent and streamlined registration processes with provisions such as pre-submission consultations, substantive guidance documents and enhanced review processes with teams of in-house reviewers and dedicated project managers, are examples of necessary prerequisites.

For developing countries such as India, international cooperation initiatives can serve as learning opportunities as well, where mature and less mature regulatory agencies collectively address issues common to all regulatory partners. India's public health demands should drive its interest and the nature of participation in international cooperation. Areas of benefit include providing expedited review pathways through international agreements in under-served disease categories, joint assessments through collaboration among regulators of countries with similar disease burdens, and the like. Although a number of harmonisation and cooperation initiatives such as the creation of single market of EU, ICH and ASEAN were initially driven by a vision to enhance trade between participating countries, the regulators' mandate to protect and promote public health makes it important to account for the public health imperative on a priority basis.

In one of the recent developments, India has joined the ranks of observers at the ICH. This is a welcome step—but India's drug regulators need to be adequately empowered within the existing policy framework, and likewise be expected to participate proactively in international forums, learn from them as well as contribute to the shaping of international processes wherever needed and possible, for their own as well as global public health.

India has arrived at the world stage—the nation's drug regulators should too!

Appendix

Table 1

Criteria for Selection of International Jurisdictions

Top 5 Countries Importing from India (2014)		*Top 5 Countries Exporting to India (2014)*	
Country	*Sum of Trade Value in USD*	*Country*	*Sum of Trade Value in USD*
USA	3761066158	USA	176254380
Russian Federation	441813171	Germany	164056658
United Kingdom	439039574	Indonesia*	108213442
South Africa	431122890	Switzerland	96220183
Nigeria	375471537	France	90919736

Note: These trade values do not reflect all pharmaceutical products that are traded (including blood products, organs, etc) but only vaccines, bulk drugs and finished formulations for therapeutic or prophylactic use.

* We have observed a discrepancy in the data for Indonesia—as per the trade data calculated from ASEAN statistics (ASEANstats, ASEAN Secretariat) for the year 2014—Indonesia's export to India amounts to USD 76,49,3496. Nonetheless, UNCOMTRADE is the only source to capture international trade data. Further, Indonesia was selected for being an interesting case study—a developing country with large local pharmaceutical industry and capacity constraint regulator.

Source: UNCOMTRADE.

Table 2

Timeline of Important Events in Pharmaceutical Regulation in India

Date	*Event*
1940	Indian Parliament passed the Drugs and Cosmetics Act, 1940, a central legislation, which regulated the sales, manufacture, distribution etc. of Drugs and Cosmetics.
1945	Drugs and Cosmetic Rules, 1945 came into being.
1948	Pharmacy Act came into being to regulate pharmacists in India.
1955	Drugs Prices Control Order, 1955 (DPCO) (under the Essential Commodities Act) came into being to regulate the drug pricing.
1988	Schedule Y was added to the Drugs and Cosmetics Rules which added set of guidelines for conducting clinical trials.
2000	The Indian Council for Medical Research or the ICMR came out with Ethical Guidelines for Biomedical Research on Human Subjects.
2001	Central Drugs Standard Control Organization (CDSCO) formed under the aegis of the Ministry of Health and Family Welfare came out with Good Clinical Practice (GCP) guidelines in compliance with the WHO and ICH guidelines.
2003	The Mashelkar Committee Report was published which recommended that offences relating to spurious drugs should be made punishable. This Report also made recommendations to change the regulatory framework present.
2005	CDSCO made changes in Schedule Y to bring it in accordance with internationally accepted norms. Schedule M of the GMP was also modified to harmonize with the WHO and US-FDA protocols.
2006	To harmonize Indian clinical trial approval process with FDA, DCGI divided all clinical trials into two categories viz.: a) trials being conducted in markets having an advanced regulatory mechanism, and b) rest of the markets. Thus, trials falling into category A did not need as much inquiry and scrutiny as those falling into category B.
2007	Clinical Trials Registry based on the WHO International Clinical Trial Registry Platform Dataset was launched, which was an online platform registering clinical trials in India.
2010	Pharmacovigilance Programme of India was launched under the aegis of CDSCO to monitor adverse drug reactions.
2013	59th Parliamentary Committee Report was published which indicted the drug regulatory authority for not implementing the Mashelkar Committee Report and made other suggestions some of which were subsequently implemented.
2013	Ministry of Health and Family Welfare constituted an expert committee under Prof Ranjit Roy Chaudhary for formulation of policies relating to drug approvals, clinical trials etc.
2013	The Drugs and Cosmetics (Amendment) Bill, 2013 was introduced in the Rajya Sabha on 29 August 2013 incorporating some of the recommendations.
31.12.2014	Another amendment Bill incorporating various changes to the present regulations was put in public domain and comments were invited from the general public.

Source: Compiled by authors.

Table 3

MoUs and Other Cooperative Agreements of US with Rest of the World

Country	*Subject*	*Effective Date*	*Expiration Date*
Australia	Pharmaceutical Good Manufacturing Practice Inspections	10-11-2000	Indefinite
Australia	Orphan Products	08/13/1997	Indefinite
Canada	Sharing and Exchange of Information about Therapeutic Products	12/01/2005	Indefinite
Canada	Drug Plan/Inspection Good Manufacturing Practices	10/01/1973	Indefinite
Canada	Good Laboratory Practices Phase I/Non-Clinical Labs	05/10/1979	Indefinite
Canada and Mexico	Scientific and Regulatory Fields of Health: Cooperation	10/30/1995	Indefinite
France	Good Laboratory Practices Phase II/Non-Clinical Labs	03/18/1986	Indefinite
Germany	Good Laboratory Practices Phase II/Non-Clinical Labs	12/23/1988	Indefinite
India	Cooperation on Medical Products	02/10/2014	02-10-2019
Japan	Good Laboratory Practices Phase I/Non-Clinical Labs	04/15/1983	Indefinite
Japan	Exchange of Good Manufacturing Practices Inspection Information	12/27/2000	Indefinite
Mexico and Canada	Scientific and Regulatory Fields of Health	10/30/1995	Indefinite
Netherlands	Good Laboratory Practices Phase II/Non-Clinical Labs	12/20/1988	Indefinite
PAHO	Regulatory Exchange Platform	05/05/2016	Indefinite
Russia	Drug Products, Good Clinical Practices	05/27/2010	Indefinite
Sweden	Good Laboratory Practices Phase I/Non-Clinical Labs	05/25/1979	Indefinite
Sweden	Drug Plant Inspections Good Manufacturing Practices; Exchange of Information	10/17/1972	Indefinite
Switzerland	Drug Plant Inspections	10/28/1968	Indefinite
Switzerland	Good Laboratory Practices Phase II/Non-Clinical Labs	04/29/1985	Indefinite
Switzerland	Drug Plant Inspections; Regulatory Cooperation	08/07/1998	Indefinite

Source: Extracted from US FDA website.

Figure 1A

Median Time to Approval for all Filed NDAs and BLAs (Months)

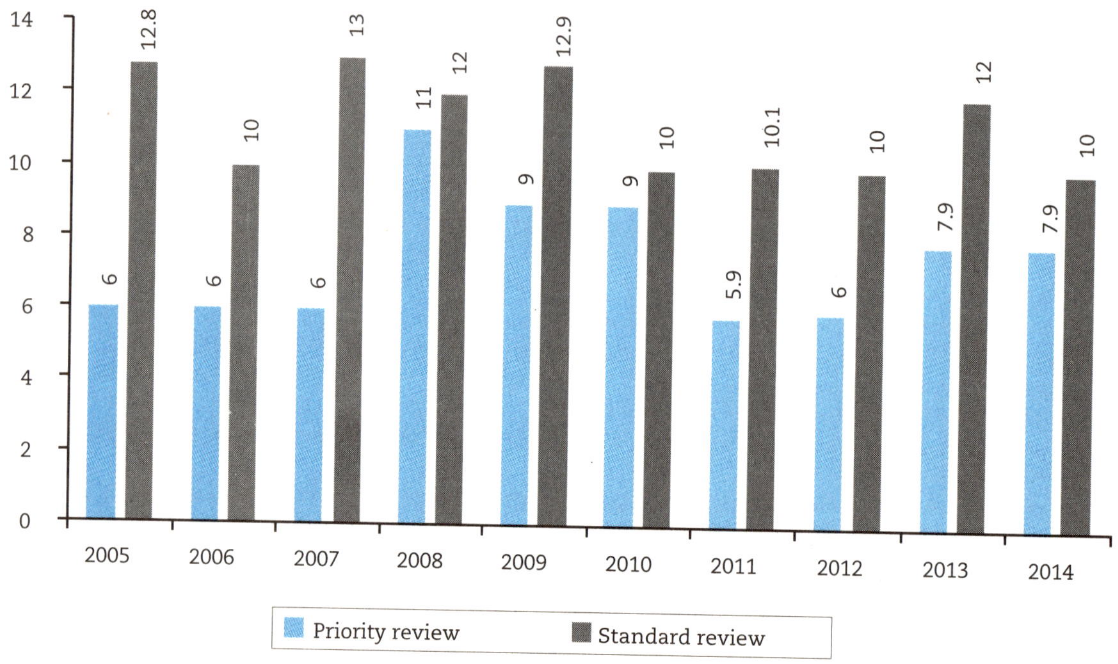

Source: FY 2015 PDUFA Performance Report, USFDA.

Bibliography

Bhatt, A. (2015). "Assessing unmet medical need in India: A regulatory riddle?", *Perspectives in Clinical Research* 6(1): 1-3. http://doi.org/10.4103/2229-3485.148786

Carpenter, D.P. (2004). "The political economy of FDA drug review: Processing, politics, and lessons for policy", *Health Affairs* 23(1): 52-63.

Chowdhury, N., P. Joshi, A. Patnaik and B. Saraswathy (2015). "Administrative structure and functions of drug regulatory authorities in India", *Working Paper* No. 309. Indian Council for Research on International Economic Relations (ICRIER).

Copland, J.R. and P. Howard (2009). *In the Wake of Wyeth V. Levine: Making the Case for Federal Preemption and Administrative Compensation*.

CIRS R&D Briefing 59 (2016). *The Impact of the Evolving Regulatory Environment on the Approval of New Medicines across Six Major Authorities 2006-2015*. Available at: *http://www.cirsci.org/wp-content/uploads/2016/05/CIRS_RD_-Briefing_59_23052016.pdf*

Dominguez-Urban, I. (1997). "Harmonization in the regulation of pharmaceutical research and human rights: The need to think globally", *Cornell International Law Journal* 30: 245.

Drezner, D.W. (2005). "Globalization, harmonization, and competition: the different pathways to policy convergence", *Journal of European Public Policy* 12(5): 841-59.

EGA Regulatory Efficiency Report (2015) Available at: *http://www.medicinesforeurope.com/wp-content/uploads/2016/03/EGA_Regulatory_Efficiency_Report_2015_low.pdf*

Imran, M., A.K. Najmi, M.F. Rashid, S. Tabrez and M.A. (2013). "Clinical research regulation in India: History, development, initiatives, challenges and controversies—Still long way to go", *Journal of Pharmacy and Bioallied Sciences* 5(1): 2

Eswaran M. and N. Gallini (2016). "Rescuing the golden age of antibiotics: can economics help avert the looming crisis?", *University of British Columbia Working Paper*. June. Available at: *http://econ.sites.olt.ubc.ca/files/2016/07/pdf_paper_eswaran_gallini-golden-age-antibiotics.pdf*. Last Accessed 9 December 2016.

Falkner, R. and A. Gupta (2009). "The limits of regulatory convergence: Globalization and GMO politics in the south", *International Environmental Agreements: Politics, Law and Economics* 9(2): 113-33.

Gray, A. (2004). *Access to Medicines and Drug Regulation in Developing Countries: A Resource Guide for DFID*. London: DFID Health Systems Resource Centre.

Hart, M. (2007). *Trading Up: The Prospect of Greater Regulatory Convergence in North America*. Mexico: International Trade and Industry Unit, Naciones Unitas CEPEL.

Hill, S. and K. Johnson (2004). *Emerging Challenges and Opportunities in Drug Registration and Regulation in Developing Countries*. Department for International Development.

Kanfer I., R.B. Walker and M.F. Skinner (2016). "South Africa", in I. Kanfer and L. Shargel (eds.), *Generic Drug Product Development: International Regulatory Requirements for Bioequivalence*. CRC Press. pp.182-210.

Katz, A. (2007). "Pharmaceutical lemons: innovation and regulation in the drug industry", *Michigan Telecommunications and Technology Law Review* 14: 1. Available online at *http://repository.law.umich.edu/cgi/viewcontent.cgi?article=1079&context=mttlr* (Accessed on 27 January 2017).

Kingham, R. and K.H. Carver (2015). "United States", in R. Kingham (ed.), *The Life Sciences Law Review*. 3rd Edition. London: Law Business Research Limited. pp.535-70.

Lakkis, M.M. (2008). "The ASEAN harmonisation scheme: Another CTD-Another challenge to the industry", *Regulatory Focus*: 39-43, November.

———. (2010). "Regulation of pharmaceutical products in Singapore", *Regulatory Focus*: 35-38. Online available at: *www.raps.org/WorkArea/DownloadAsset.aspx?id=3224* (Accessed on 15 January 2017).

Lee, C.E. and K. Satku (eds.) (2015). "Singapore's health care system: What 50 years have achieved", *World Scientific*.

Leng, H.M., D. Sanders and A.P. Pollock (2015). "Pro-generics policies and the backlog in medicines registration in South Africa: Implications for access to essential and affordable medicines", in *GaBI J* 4(2): 58-63.

Leng, H.M., A.M. Pollock and D. Sanders (2016). "The impact of the Medicines Control Council backlog and fast-track review system on access to innovative and new generic and biosimilar medicines of public health importance in South Africa", *SAMJ: South African Medical Journal* 106(4): 350-53.

Lezotre, P.L. (2014). *International Cooperation, Convergence and Harmonisation of Pharmaceutical Regulations: A Global Perspective*. Academic Press.

Liberti, L., N. McAuslane and P. Patel (2012). *Characterising the Influencers of Submission Lag Time for Medicines in the Emerging Markets: Analysis of Short and Long Lag Time Factors*. The Centre for Innovation in Regulatory Science.

Lustig, T.A. and V. Weisfeld (eds.) (2013). *International Regulatory Harmonization amid Globalization of Drug Development: Workshop Summary*. National Academies Press. Available from: *http://www.ncbi.nlm.nih.gov/books/NBK174226/* (Accessed on 15 October 2016).

Lutter, R. and D. Zorn (2016). "Improving regulatory cooperation between US Food and Drug Administration and the EU", *Working Paper*. Washington, DC: The George Washington University Regulatory Studies Center. Retrieved 6 September 2016, from *https://regulatorystudies.columbian.gwu.edu/sites/regulatorystudies.columbian.gwu.edu/files/downloads/Lutter-Zorn_Improving-Cooperation-FDA-EU_WP.pdf*

Matsebula, T., J. Goudge and L. Gilson (2005). "Regulating the pharmaceutical sector: Coping with low capacity while maintaining regulatory independence", in *Health Economics Financing Programme (HEFP) Working Paper* 1(05).

Mehdi, A., D. Chaudhry, P. Tomar and P. Joshi (2016). "Prevention of chronic diseases: Reorienting primary health systems in India", *Indian Council for Research on International Economic Relations (ICRIER), Working Paper* No. 321.

Meyer, B.D. (1995). "Natural and quasi-experiments in economics", *Journal of business & economic statistics* 13(2): 151-61.

Parsons, A., W. Allison, M. Justin, K. Liesel and R. Lake (2015). "South Africa", in R. Kingham (ed.), *The Life Sciences Law Review*. 3rd Edition. London: Law Business Research Limited. pp.451-66.

Pettman, S. (2013). "Standards harmonisation in ASEAN: Progress, challenges and moving beyond 2015", *ERIA Discussion Paper Series* (30).

Philipson, T. and E. Sun (2010). *Cost of Caution: The Impact on Patients of Delayed Drug Approvals*. Project FDA Report (2). New York: The Manhattan Institute for Policy Research.

Puig-Junoy, J. (2005). *The Public Financing of Pharmaceuticals*. Edward Elgar Publishing.

Ratanawijitrasin, S. (2007). *Drug Regulation and Incentives for Innovation: The Case of ASEAN*. WHO. Available at: *www.who.int/intellectualproperty/studies/Drugregulationincentives.pdf*

Raymond, A.S. and A.J. Humphreys (2013). "Human medicinal products in the European Union: Procedures", in J.P. Griffin, J. Posner and G. R. Barker (eds.), *The Textbook of Pharmaceutical Medicine*. 7th edition. London: Wiley Blackwell.

———. (2013). "Human medicinal products in the European Union: Regulations directives and structures", in John P. Griffin, John Posner, Geoffrey R. Barker (eds.), *The Textbook of Pharmaceutical Medicine.* 7th edition. London: Wiley Blackwell.

Sangai et al. (2016). *Pharmaceutical Regulation and Public Health Need, in Law in Numbers: Evidence-based Approaches to Legal Reform.* Vidhi-Centre for Legal Policy

Speers, S., V. Benton and S. Rose (2016). "Challenges and opportunities in the ASEAN emerging regulatory landscape", *Regulatory Rapporteur* 13(3), March.

Stephanou, C.A. (2003). "Regulatory convergence in the wider Europe region: Goals and means", *Working Paper* No. 1. *https://www.ause.eu/public/medias/2003_1_2003_CA_STEPHANOU.pdf* (Accessed on 10 January 2017).

Swann, G.P. (2010). "International standards and trade: A review of the empirical literature", *OECD Trade Policy Working Papers*, No. 97. OECD Publishing. doi: 10.1787/5kmdbg9xktwg-en

TACD (2001). *Briefing Paper on Mutual Recognition Agreements. http://test.tacd.org/wp-content/uploads/2013/09/TACD-TRADE-2001-Briefing-Paper-on-Mutual-Recognition-Agreements.pdf*

Venkateswarlu, B., D. Nagarjuna, M. Ramaiah, M. Nagabhushanam and M.V. Akram (2014). "Regulatory requirements for the registration of generic Solid Orals in USA, Singapore, Malaysia, and Thailand", *Journal of Global Trends in Pharmaceutical Sciences*: 5(4): 2225-32.

Vishwanath T.S. (2016). "A blueprint for harmonized markets &trade links", in T.T. Yong. and A. Bhattacharya (ed.), *Looking Ahead: India & Singapore in the New Millennium.* ISAS-NUS & Ananta Aspen Centre, Baskerville BT, Lustra Print Process Pvt. Ltd. pp.75-83.

Vogel, D. (1998). "The globalization of pharmaceutical regulation", *Governance* 11(1): 1-22.

Wong, E. (2003). "The regulatory environment and clinical trials in Southeast Asia", *Drug Information Journal* 37(4): 155-64.